Natural Health after Birth

"Thirty years ago, when I had my babies, we were rediscovering natural birth and breast-feeding. But, we struggled alone during postpartum. If I had been able to read Aviva's book then, I would have cried less. Every new mother should have a copy of this book."

PEGGY O'MARA,
EDITOR AND PUBLISHER
OF *MOTHERING* MAGAZINE

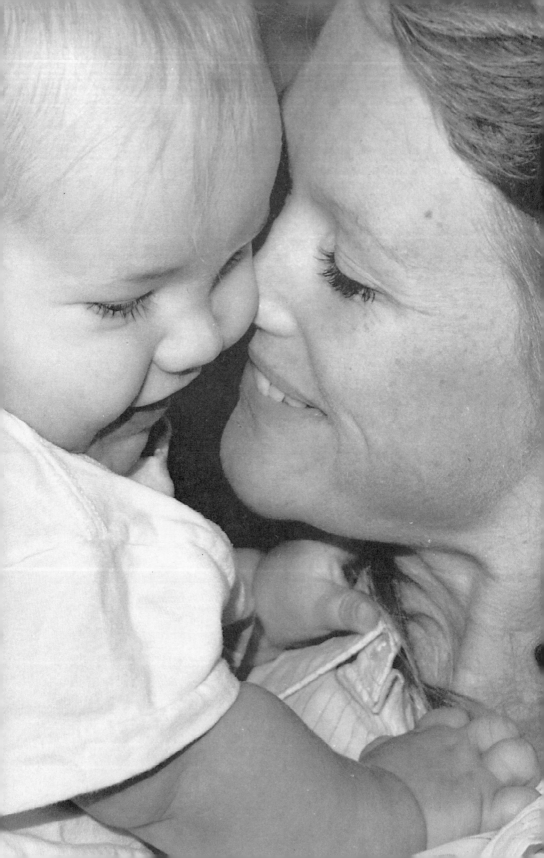

Natural Health after Birth

The Complete Guide to Postpartum Wellness

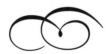

AVIVA JILL ROMM

Healing Arts Press
Rochester, Vermont

Healing Arts Press
One Park Street
Rochester, Vermont 05767
www.InnerTraditions.com

Healing Arts Press is a division of Inner Traditions International

Note to the reader: This book is intended as an informational guide. The remedies, approaches, and techniques described herein are meant to supplement, and not to be a substitute for, professional medical care or treatment. They should not be used to treat a serious ailment without prior consultation with a qualified health care professional.

Library of Congress Cataloging-in-Publication Data
Romm, Aviva Jill.
    Natural health after birth : the complete guide to postpartum wellness / Aviva Jill Romm.
      p. cm.
    Includes bibliographical references and index.
    ISBN 0-89281-930-8
1. Postnatal care. 2. Motherhood. 3. Yoga. 4. Naturopathy. I. Title.
RG801 .R65 2002
618.6—dc21   2001051649

Printed and bound in the United States

10 9 8 7 6 5 4 3 2 1

Text design and layout by Priscilla Baker
This book was typeset in Caslon with Koch Antiqua as a display typeface

Yoga posture photographs of Aviva Romm on pages 221–24 by Jay Land
Chapter opening photographs by Suzanne Arms

Dedication

To my beautiful children—Iyah, Yemima, Forest, and Naomi—who love me regardless of the fact that I keep writing books, who have grown so beautiful that every day of my life is filled with continual awe, and who are my best friends and teachers. You are my beloveds forever.

To my husband, Tracy Romm, who took such loving care of me after each of our babies was born, who takes care of me as each book is born, and who is rock solid in my life.

To Kim Land, Sarahn Henderson, and Lisa Olko, who were also there after my babies were born, and who have been here ever since. And to Lizzie McDaniels Feigenbaum, who began this journey with me and who continues it with me ever steady. May deep satisfaction and joy be yours, and may your families be blessed with strength and love.

To the midwives, herbalists, and docs who are my friends, teachers, and companions in this work we are blessed to do. It is truly a pleasure to share this road with each of you. Our passions and our hearts meet in sacred places and I am honored to know each of you as part of my family. Thanks especially to Roy Upton, David Winston, Andy Ellis, and Lesley and Michael Tierra for information on Native American and traditional Chinese postpartum care traditions.

To my mom, Wendy, and my grandma Ida, who welcomed me into the world and who love me still.

To Jon Graham and Lee Juvan, my editors at Healing Arts Press: Jon, who helped this book get its start; and Lee, who put up with me with endless faith as I kept extending past my deadline . . . and to Lee's family, which grew to include her first baby as this book was nearing completion (I got it done for your postpartum, at least, eh?).

And to all of the families who have let me into the secret, magical, hard, and joyous places of their lives. You have shaped who I am.

I love the infinite light within each of you.

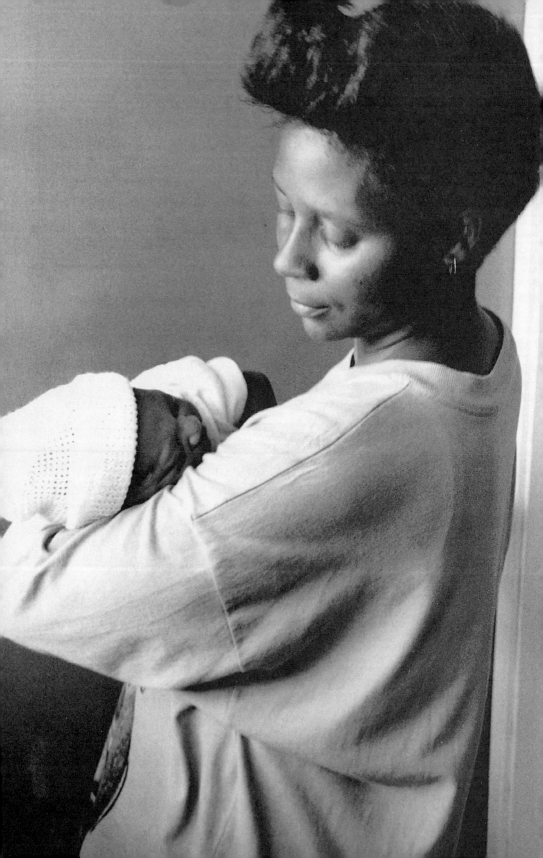

Contents

THREE

Preparing for the Postpartum Before Baby Is Born • 61

FOUR

The First Days after Birth • 83

FIVE

The Next Six Weeks • 131

SIX

Nutrition for New Mothers • 177

SEVEN

Into the First Year • 195

EIGHT

Replenishing Yourself: Body, Mind, and Spirit • 213

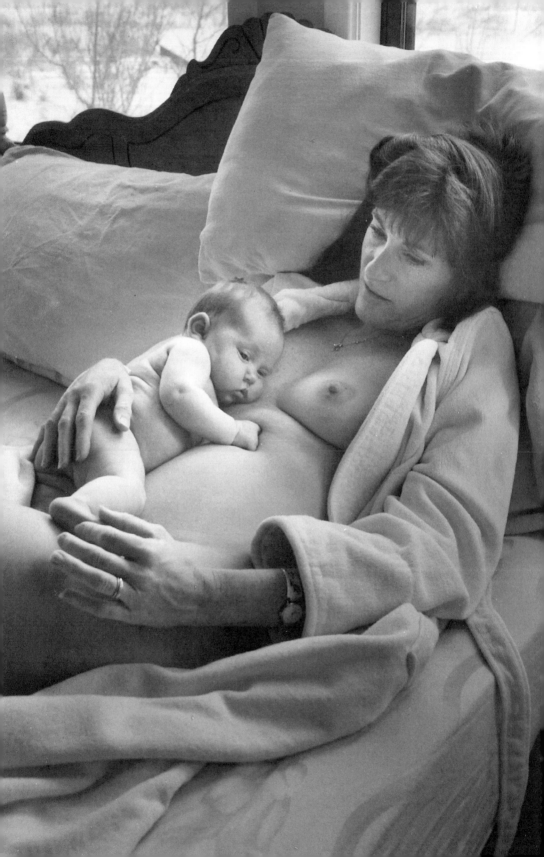

Introduction

Circles

The moon is most happy when it is full
And the sun always looks like a perfectly minted gold coin that was just
Placed in flight
By God's playful kiss
And so many varieties of fruit hang plump and round from
Branches that seem like a sculptor's hands
I see the beautiful curve of a pregnant belly
Shaped by a soul within
And the earth itself and the planets and the spheres
I have gotten a hint
There is something about circles the beloved likes.

Hafiz

A woman is the full circle, within her is the power—to create,
nurture, and transform.

Diane Marieschild

*Y*ou haven't had a full night's sleep in 6 weeks (or has it been 6 months?), you weigh 15 pounds more than you'd like to and still don't fit into your favorite jeans, your sex life seems to have gone out the window, and you haven't dusted your house in longer than you care to remember. Your girlfriend from work stops by and, after telling you how cute the baby is, fills you in on all the gossip from work as well as on the business accounts you handed over to her while taking an extended maternity leave without pay so you could be home with your precious baby. Your precious baby is now crying because your girlfriend's visit interfered with his nap—and yours—and you are exhausted, too. After she leaves, you break down crying along with the baby. As you sink onto your bed to nurse him, you feel confused about your new role, what you're missing by being home full time,

1

and whether it's all worth it. You feel lost and out of touch with the adult world.

Yet as your baby begins to nurse, his crying stops and he looks up into your eyes, a smile playing at the corner of his lips as he desperately tries to keep nursing while communicating his love to you. Soon his eyes drift backward in sleep, and you melt at his beauty and pure sweetness. You begin to relax, remember why you chose to be home with your baby, and, picking up a book to read, feel the bliss of motherhood sweep over you. You, too, soon drift off to sleep, grateful for these precious moments with your child. Sound familiar? It's postpartum!

The time after birth is known as the *postpartum* or *postnatal* period—both terms meaning "after birth." Medical texts define *postpartum* as the 6-week period of time from after the birth of the baby until a woman's reproductive organs have returned to their nonpregnant condition. However, this definition is too limited. It ignores the fact that it takes much longer than 6 weeks to heal from giving birth, and much longer than this to adjust to the momentous experience of becoming a mother.

This is a time of enormous physical, emotional, psychological, and spiritual growth and change for women (and men), whether or not this is your first child. It's also a time of great emotional ups and downs and conflicting feelings. Each passage through birth and into motherhood is a journey into the unknown, with new hopes, fears, expectations, and demands. Although newborns are doted on with kisses, praise, and gifts, most women receive little special attention and nurturing during this time, leaving many new mothers to doubt whether they're up to the task when they feel stressed, exhausted, or overwhelmed in spite of the sweet and adorable bundle they hold in their arms. And many mothers—most, in fact—feel isolated in the experience of motherhood, wondering if they're the only ones who think they're coming apart at the seams. Factors such as a difficult or disappointing birth, financial worries, and an unsupportive environment can compound stress, anxiety, and a sense of aloneness.

Defining the postpartum as a finite period of 6 weeks leads many new mothers to feel as if they're taking too long to "get it together," or that they're overwhelmed by something that shouldn't be such a big deal. It also leads many women to go without help and support too quickly after birth, and to return to work outside the home before they are emotionally or physically ready. Societal expectations also revolve around this arbitrarily allotted

6-week period. Many employers expect women to be back to their old selves after 6 weeks, the obstetrician's and midwife's care packages end at 6 weeks, and even husbands, other relatives, and friends expect Mom to be able to cope on her own by then.

Yet most women, when given the opportunity to express their intimate feelings about the time after birth, say they needed more help, support, care, guidance, and understanding than they received, and for much longer than 6 weeks after giving birth. Most mothers say they don't really begin to feel like their old selves for 6 to 8 months after birth, and many never feel quite like their old selves again, their lives having been permanently (and usually beautifully) transformed by this new being in their lives. Most admit they had feelings of profound joy as well as stress, anxiety, and confusion during those early days, weeks, and months of new motherhood.

Furthermore, family systems aren't what they used to be. In some families, traditional roles still exist: Mothers and fathers live together, the father assumes the role of primary breadwinner, and the mother assumes full responsibility for childcare. But this model has, for better or worse, been joined by additional family models ranging from two-parent, two-income homes; to stay-at-home dads with Mom earning the money; to single-mother and single-father households. Each model presents its own stresses on the family, and each poses unique postpartum dilemmas and considerations. Increasingly, mothers share the responsibility for bringing in an income while maintaining primary responsibility for the children. Fortunately, more fathers now get involved, but the multiplicity of roles today's women face as they become mothers has dramatically increased the pressures felt by childbearing women. Due to the complexity of family structures, and because this book focuses on the needs of women after birth, I have addressed the book toward women. However, fathers, care providers, and family members and friends of childbearing women will all derive from this book information and insights that can be used to provide support for the new mothers in their lives.

Additionally, I refer to birth partners as fathers, trusting that those in this role other than the father, or other than a male, can replace *father* with the appropriate noun or pronoun to reflect their own situation. Women having babies as a couple, single moms with support partners other than the father, and so on will, I hope, forgive my using this convention for the sake of simplicity. Please know that you have been equally included in my thoughts as I have written this book. An intimate and caring support person is a tremendous source of encouragement and inspiration for a new mother. When this person is the life partner, he, too, is likely to be going through great personal transformation. Thus, I have included thoughts for fathers, too.

Though many fathers have confided their own fears and anxieties over the years, my perspective is still that of a woman, and the intensity of postnatal experience lies not only within the psychological change of becoming a parent, but also in the dramatic physical transformation of the pregnant body to the nonpregnant body—a phenomenon germane only to the female of our species. Therefore, my primary focus here is on the needs of new mothers. I do hope men who are taking a more active role in parenting begin to talk and publish more about the transformation to fatherhood, and will encourage increasing numbers of men to participate in the childbearing experience as intimate friends to their wives. It is also my hope that our social institutions will shift toward a model of shared responsibility for childbearing, thus putting in place the benefits that will enable parents to do this.

As a midwife and a mother of four children, I have both witnessed and experienced the births of numerous babies. I have been privileged to be included in the intimate experience of women becoming mothers. I know firsthand both the intense and the indescribable joy of watching a baby unfold before my eyes from the cocoon of the womb in the minutes and hours after birth; I have felt the surge of joy fill my heart as I looked into the profound depth of my new baby's eyes, smelled the pure delicious scent of my baby's soft skin, and sighed with my husband in near disbelief that we were so blessed to have each beautiful child who has graced our home. I have also felt the tumultuous range of emotions and physical sensations that accompany those early days, weeks, and months as a woman and her family adjust physically, emotionally, and socially to a new baby. And like many other mothers these days, I wanted to care for my baby and myself naturally, without unnecessary medical interventions, chemical applications, and synthetic substances. Now, with my oldest child 16 years old and my youngest seven years old, I wonder where the time went, and wish, in moments of stress and chaos, I had only known how quickly it would fly. All of the years we have with our children are magical and special, but those early days when we set the foundations of trust and tenderness are all too precious. Were there only more resources available to make those days easier emotionally, to validate my experience of feeling torn between the important work of motherhood and my personal needs, reminding me that being a mother is important and irreplaceable work, and that time does, indeed, pass all too quickly.

This book is a resource of support, natural treatments, and best-kept herbal treasures for new mothers. It is a source of validation and inspiration for women experiencing the ups and downs of becoming mothers—the joys and hardships, the physical changes, the elation and depression, the euphoria and exhaustion. In other words, this book is for all new mothers! While many birth and postpartum books focus on caring for the new baby, this one is all about the needs of new mothers. Of course, all new mothers are concerned about the health and safety of their babies; and there are numerous excellent references to describe the changes and needs of healthy newborns. But there are few books that focus on the needs of the woman in her growing role as mother.

Women reading this book prenatally will gain a clear sense of how best to prepare for the postpartum so that their transition to motherhood is as smooth and joyful as possible. New mothers reading this book will gain a greater understanding of what they are going through and how best to get their needs met while themselves meeting the needs of their new and growing family. And mothers reading *Natural Health after Birth* late in the first year after the birth of their first baby—and those preparing for the births of subsequent babies—I hope will sigh a sigh, shed a tear, and break into a smile as they recognize their own feelings within the pages of this book.

Arranged chronologically, this book takes you through the first two years of life after giving birth. It is my desire that this book will support women in feeling whole as they embrace motherhood. This is really my prayer for society. Whole women make happier mothers. Happier mothers make happier babies. Happier babies grow into healthier children and adults, and thus we see how the care a woman receives after birth sows the seeds for a healthier society.

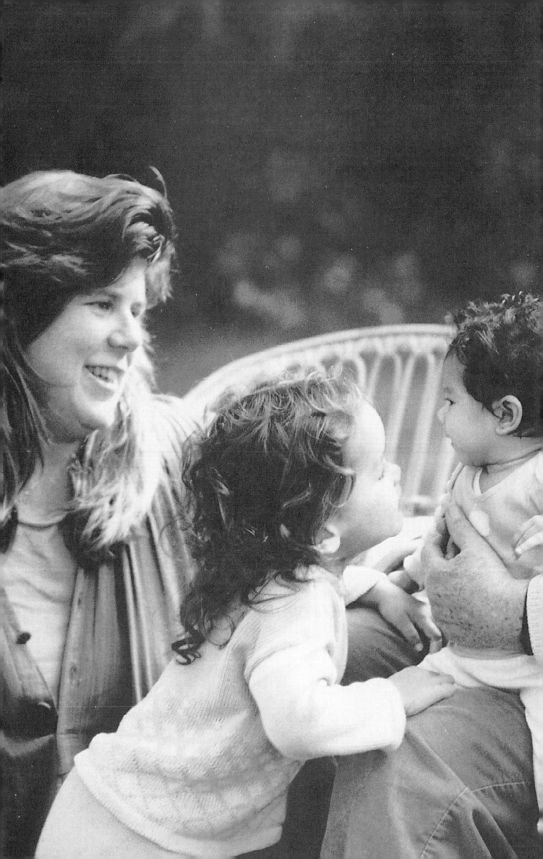

ONE

The Birth of a Mother

Women who become mothers find that it is often in the crucible
of that experience, in what in so many ways seems a sacrifice of
self, that she touches her deepest experience of the female self
and wrestles with an angel that at once wounds and blesses her.
Naomi Ruth Lowinsky, ***Stories from the Motherline***

M atrescence is a term coined by anthropologist Dana Raphael in her book *The Tender Gift: Breastfeeding* to describe the process of becoming a mother, compared to adolescence, the process of becoming an adult. Matrescence begins in earnest when we become pregnant, and continues until the day arrives when we realize we finally feel like a mom, steady on our feet after the roller coaster of emotions and demands of those first months after birth. Matrescence requires patience, nurturing, support, and understanding, both from ourselves and from our family and community. It also requires an inner determination to embrace motherhood as part of our personal identity.

❧ BIRTH: ONLY THE BEGINNING ❧

"We have come a long way in our understanding of birth, its physiology, psychology, and spirituality. The birth experience is recognized as a rite of passage for all involved," says Sylvia Reichman in *Mothering* magazine. "But what about afterwards, when the birth experience has taken its place as a part of life and there is the new mom, alone with her new baby?" she asks. In cultures where rites of passage are a significant and transformative life experience, a period of integration generally follows. This is the time during which the initiate, in this case the mother, assimilates the experience—the birth of her child—and her new role in the community. This integration period may include ceremony, celebration, time to tell the story of the rite of passage, and other forms of honoring and doting. Yet in our society little, if anything, is done for the new mother after birth to honor, celebrate, and support her as she integrates her new identity and role as a mother. Nor is she provided time simply to enjoy the precious and fleeting period when her child is a newborn.

When a person goes through a rite of passage in a traditional culture, and is initiated into a new phase of life—for example, a young woman emerging into adult status—the experienced members of that particular group pass on to the initiate their secrets and the pearls of wisdom gathered from years of experience. The initiate is often assisted in assuming the new role through instruction, apprenticeship, or another form of guidance.

In our culture there is little preparation, either before or after birth, for the tremendous changes that we as women will experience as we become mothers, and little recognition that the rite of passage of birth does not end the minute the baby is born. Indeed, those early months after the birth should be considered an extension of the rite of passage of birth. Yet most childbirth classes fail to adequately prepare women and men for the rigors of parenthood in those early months, focusing mainly on the upcoming birth, and many people are so preoccupied by the imminence of the birth that they are unable to take in much about life after birth.

However, birth—though it is quite dramatic due to the physical, emotional, and spiritual intensity of the experience—is only a doorway that connects the process of *becoming* a mother to that of *caring for* a child for a lifetime. We tend to see birth as the culmination of all that our pregnancy preparation is intended for. Once the birth has been accomplished and the mother and baby are considered "out of the woods," it is generally expected that Mom can recover quickly and get on with life, blissful in the glow of motherhood. Early hospital discharge may reinforce for those in the mother's intimate circle that she has been given the medical seal of approval and that she has, indeed, recovered. However, this is far from the truth. Women who have just given birth are physically open and emotionally vulnerable for weeks—even months—after they have given birth.

❧ WHAT IS THE POSTPARTUM? ☙

Midwife Raven Lang once said, "As long as the baby is still in diapers and you're up in the night, you're postpartum." Such a view reminds women that the demands of motherhood—including intense sleep deprivation and maximum amounts of energy being poured out 24 hours a day, 7 days a week to another person—no matter how loved and wanted that baby is, are draining. Unfortunately, our cultural definition of postpartum does not include Lang's more simple and holistic view.

In medical lingo, the postpartum, also called the postnatal period or the *puerperium,* is the 6 weeks from the time of the birth until the woman is no longer considered an obstetric patient. What is respected as a precious and sacred time for women in many cultures around the world has been defined in Western clinical medical terms as follows: "The puerperium is the period of a few weeks that starts immediately after delivery and is completed when the reproductive tract has returned anatomically to the normal nonpregnant condition. Although the changes occurring during this period are physiologic, in few, if any, other circumstances are there such marked and rapid metabolic events in the absence of disease." (Pritchard and Macdonald 1976)

This dry passage, taken from the still-taught classic medical textbook *Williams Obstetrics,* as well as the rest of the chapter on postpartum care found in that book, defines the postpartum experience solely on the basis of the physical changes that occur in the reproductive tract. No mention is made of the tremendous emotional impact these physical changes have on the woman, nor is the psychological, social, emotional, or spiritual experience of the mother ever mentioned. It is acknowledged, however, that the postnatal period is a time of unparalleled change in the otherwise healthy human body.

The classic text *Nurse-Midwifery* reiterates the above narrow medical definition with an added grim emphasis on the permanent nature of the physical changes a woman experiences:

> The postpartal period is the period of time from the delivery of the placenta and membranes . . . to the return of the woman's reproductive tract to its nonpregnant condition. Note that this is to the nonpregnant, not prepregnant, condition as is often said erroneously. The prepregnant condition is gone forever—the most strikingly so after the first pregnancy and childbirth experience but also true with each subsequent experience in relation to the prepregnant state of the organs each time.
>
> The puerperium lasts approximately six weeks. (Varney 1980)

To the credit of midwives, a discussion of the potential for emotional and social upheaval in the new mother's life does ensue in this text, emphasizing the physiologic as well as emotional basis of postpartum depression and grief. Yet several implicit messages are embedded in these passages that actually contribute to the level of care, or lack thereof, that women receive in the days, weeks, and months after they birth, directly influencing the nature of American women's postpartum experiences. The primary message women receive is that they are merely going through physical changes; secondary is the message that they will never be "themselves" again. Women are told at their postpartum-care visits that their aches and complaints are "normal," the "baby blues" are a natural part of postpartum recovery, and just to "give it time." However, according to Varney, they may never feel "back to their old selves" again. The notion that a woman's pre-pregnant identity is gone forever is not only a terrifying idea for childbearing women, but is also not entirely true. As a new mother there are definitely times when your identity has been subsumed by motherhood, but in the long run, as a mother you expand your identity, not lose it.

While newborns receive no shortage of attention, new mothers are rarely asked how they're feeling emotionally, how they're coping with the changes they experience, whether they're getting help around the house or what they need. Yet we are somehow expected magically to be recovered at 6 weeks postpartum. This is most vividly reflected in the fact that few employers are tolerant of maternity leave that extends beyond this 6-week period, and in this country paternity leave of even 6 weeks is virtually unheard of. A woman who wants a longer maternity leave often must take it without pay.

The fact that women no longer are considered obstetric patients after 6 weeks also reflects the belief that women are expected to be physically recovered enough to resume their previous responsibilities. This causes women to place unfair expectations on themselves, and may also lead their mates to have unrealistic expectations that Mom can "handle it all," just as she perhaps did before baby. Indeed, most women begin to resume their responsibilities within a week or two of the birth, trying to be back in full swing by 6 weeks postpartum. For moms with more than one child, this may mean running an older sibling back and forth to playgroup or school, going grocery shopping, doing the housecleaning, preparing for meals, and caring for baby. And for a mom with a job outside the home (or who works from home), whether or not she has other children, this may mean doing all of this in addition to a full- or part-time career.

Finally, and perhaps most significantly, the 6-week time defined by the term *postpartum period* relates only to the physical recovery of the mom from birth, relegating the profound experience of birth and motherhood to a physical, medical phenomenon, thereby denying the enormous human significance of the transformation. Women themselves may feel energetic and exuberant enough at 6 weeks postpartum to get back into the swing of things, only to wonder why they are exhausted by 7 P.M., why they are having renewed postpartum bleeding, why they cry at a critical comment made by their mother-in-law, friend, or boss, why they snap at their toddler for spilling a cup of juice, or why they don't feel like having a sexual relationship with their husband.

Many new mothers feel a profound and even surprising sense of identification with other mothers in the world, and with this may come an increased sense of urgency about international political unrest, violence in their community, or environmental hazards that are perceived as a threat not only to their own children, but also to other children worldwide. For many women, becoming a mother opens a well of transpersonal sensitivity that extends far beyond anything that can be reduced to physical changes, no matter how complex and dramatic these may be.

❧ POSTNATAL CARE ☙

In *Reactions to Motherhood: The Role of Post-Natal Care*, midwife Jean A. Ball writes: "The main focus of postnatal care has traditionally been that of ensuring the physical recovery of the mother from the effects of pregnancy and labor and establishing infant feeding patterns. . . . The emotional and psychological needs of mothers have not received much attention until recently and there has been an assumption that these needs will automatically be met if the first two aspects of care are satisfied. The organization of postnatal care has accordingly been based upon this premise." Interestingly, recent studies question the effectiveness of postpartum medical visits in meeting the postpartum health needs of mothers, and conclude that "the present six week postnatal examination does not appear to meet the health needs of women after childbirth: its content and timing should be reviewed" (Bick and MacArthur 1995).

According to noted childbirth author Sheila Kitzinger, "The postnatal check-up usually takes place six weeks after the birth. It is difficult to understand why it occurs then, not earlier or later. Indeed, it is questionable why it needs to be done routinely, except that some women might be so busy with the baby that they put off seeking medical help though they really need it. . . . In modern technological cultures the medical system controls the gateway to motherhood and has devised its own rituals, so that a woman might not feel safe if she does not attend her postnatal check-up though she is completely fit" (Kitzinger 1994). Placksin remarks that postpartum time frames, be they 3 days, 2 weeks, or 6 weeks, are arbitrary, and don't reflect anything but events in medical care—for example, at 3 days the milk comes in or baby may become jaundiced; at 2 weeks the baby goes for a pediatric visit; at 6 weeks you have your final postpartum exam at the doctor's or midwife's office.

A study published in *Midwifery* states, "Women are prepared to attend postnatal assessments but may have examinations without obvious reason, while other tests which might be helpful for certain conditions are infrequently used. Substantial postpartum morbidity [health problems] is known to exist and this is not routinely assessed at the postnatal assessment" (Bick and MacArthur 1995).

"In a study of 11,701 postpartum women, nearly half had health problems within three months after the birth which continued for more than 6 weeks, and which they never experienced before. The symptoms of ill health which they confronted sometimes lasted for months or years afterward, and many of them never told their doctors about them" (MacArthur, Lewis, and Knox 1991—see notes from Kitzinger). In general, the medical community, and the cursory nature of postnatal care, does not facilitate the intimacy of relationship from which women might express the nature of their physical complaints and has not recognized the extent to which women experience health complaints. Furthermore, a thorough look at the medical literature reveals that although there are high rates of discomfort and physical health problems for postpartum women, little attention has been given to research in this area beyond recent studies of postpartum depression.

According to Kitzinger and others, postpartum visits should focus on the challenges women face during this time, and should provide women with the opportunity to express their concerns and expectations, both physically and emotionally. According to a study by Buchart and colleagues from the Department of Nursing at the University of Cape Town, "Listening to women is an essential element in the provision of flexible and responsive postnatal care that meets the felt needs of women and their families" (Buchart et al. 1999). Only by asking women how they feel can their felt needs be known.

Midwives, often mothers themselves, have the perfect opportunity to provide new mothers with meaningful care and attention in the postnatal period—and many recognize the significance of this time. By developing an open dialogue with new mothers, midwives can help women to prepare realistically for the postpartum prior to birth, encouraging them to line up support for both their physical and emotional well-being. And while few—if any—midwives have the time to move in with their clients for a week after birth as midwives often did even up until 100 years ago, they can make it clear that they have the time and interest to value your postpartum recovery as much as they did your prenatal and birth wellness.

During the postpartum, the midwife may visit you in your home, or encourage you to come into the office with baby for "tea and a chat" as often as you need to. Provided with a comfortable and supportive environment and a willing listener, you as the new mother may feel secure enough to confide your inner feelings and thoughts, as well as discuss physical discomforts or areas of concern. In my own practice, as part of my routine childbearing services, I visit the new family on the first and fourth days after the birth, then at 2 and 6 weeks encourage visits back at my office. In addition, I speak to new mothers and fathers daily in the first week, and several times a week thereafter. My birthing services include postpartum care through the first 3 months after birth at no additional charge, regardless of how many visits or phone contacts my clients require. When interviewing care providers for pregnancy and birth, be sure to ask them what kind of postnatal care you are entitled to, and what this includes. Your need for care and support will not end at the birth, nor will your health-related questions. Having someone available to you for 3 months postpartum can be an important part of your healthcare plan.

ꙮ THE FOURTH TRIMESTER ꙮ

Rather than limiting postpartum to an arbitrary 6 weeks, many midwives, childbirth educators, and postpartum doulas are encouraging women to see the postpartum as a fourth trimester, thus allowing themselves *at least* a full 3 months for physical recovery, spiritual integration, and emotional assimilation. Even 3 months, many experts agree, may be too short a time. Many mothers say it was closer to 8 months before they began to feel more settled in their role as mother, and able also to regain a sense of personal identity and clarity. Three months, however, may be considered the first milestone when women begin to feel like they are getting their feet on the ground. It also gives friends and family a clear framework for setting expectations for the mother, allowing her 3 full months to receive active help and support. Most of all, it allows her to be gentle with herself on those days that are more challenging, and gives her an excuse to lie around snuggling with that beautiful baby, savoring every minute as he or she blossoms before her eyes.

After the 3-month milestone, you can realistically expect to continue to experience emotional peaks and valleys for many more months as hormones fluctuate, eating habits vary, sleep deprivation continues, baby breast-feeds, and you strive to keep up with the baby's changing schedule and needs. As a midwife I continue to get calls from mothers well into the first year after they've given birth, with questions about sleeping habits, teething, breast feeding, introducing solid foods, and so on. It's always an opportunity to really check in with the mom to see how she's doing, whether she's caring for herself as well as she's caring for her baby, and to praise her on a job well done. These phone conversations are often filled with sighs of relief from the moms as they hear me remind them that feeling overwhelmed is part of the territory of motherhood in our fast-paced society, and reflects no short-comings of their own. Expanding the definition of postpartum to include the first year after birth may initially seem like a long time, which in itself may be intimidating, but in the long run it allows you flexible boundaries and should relieve you of a false deadline that says you have to "have it together" by a certain time.

⊱ SIGNS AND GUIDEPOSTS ⊰

Although you need to be flexible and think big in terms of your personal definition of how long the postpartum period should last, allowing yourself to think of the postpartum as a finite but flexible period will help you feel more confident that the postpartum is not interminable. Knowing you are experiencing tumultuous emotions and hectic days because you are in the midst of a unique phase of your life, rather than in a permanent situation, can be most reassuring and comforting, especially on the days when you wonder if it will always be like this now that you are a mom. Some women feel they can't remember what life was like before baby, and are afraid they'll never feel like their familiar, competent selves again. Others wonder if there will always be more work and stress piled on top of what they are already doing. Realistic expectations and time frames are thus essential to help you keep perspective on what you might be experiencing.

The best time frames, signs, and guideposts, however, may not come from medical professionals but instead from mothers themselves, who can share with you how they have felt at various stages during the first year after birth. According to Sally Placksin, "Women don't have a universal language to describe this time and create internal maps on false recovery time periods. . . . Women need navigational guideposts of physical and emotional changes and they need companionship and role models." It is important to remember, though, that every woman is different, and some will integrate motherhood faster than others. Therefore, it is important to speak with several mothers and create a sort of composite expectation.

There are certain common experiences of motherhood that we all share—for example, the emotional fluctuations we feel as our milk comes in, the anxiety we feel during the first days we are home alone with our newborns, the sleepless nights, the frustration we feel when our babies are 6 months old and we feel like we should really have it together by then but we don't, the smiles, the tears. Sheila Kitzinger reminds us that while certain postpartum realities are nearly universal, how we interpret them varies. Studies of mothers reveal that at least half of all mothers in Western society feel inadequate or guilty much of the time. We must be as gentle and patient with ourselves as we wish to be with our babies.

Other women's experiences can be a valuable frame of reference for you, serving as a reminder that you are not alone, not crazy, and not incompetent. However, remember that you, too, will be different, and must honor what you bring to the story. Just as some children learn to walk at 8 months and others at 14 months, so too do mothers begin to stand on their own feet in their own time. It's important for mothers to remember, even when their children are well into their teens, that they don't have to have it together all the time or know all the answers.

❧ HONORING OUR RANGE OF EMOTIONS ❧

New motherhood has the potential to bring with it the entire range of human emotions—from unimaginable bliss and joy, to grief, rage, and resentment. Unfortunately, deeply ingrained, unrealistic cultural stereotypes of the perfect mother—independent, competent, able to handle a multitude of tasks simultaneously, self-sacrificing, and happy—may make you feel entirely unfit for your new responsibilities. Pregnancy brings with it a heightened sense of awareness, both physically and emotionally, which is only intensified by loss of sleep, dramatic hormonal changes, and incredible demands on your nutrition if you are breast-feeding. We come face to face with many aspects of our personality, finding ourselves more tender and nurturing toward another human being than we have ever imagined, and more out of control than we might dare to admit. You may find yourself struggling simply to figure out how to find time to grab a shower and fix a snack with a newborn to look after, or you might harbor secret thoughts of abandoning your whole family and running away to a quiet place. Most mothers, until the baby is at least 6 weeks old—and frequently older—feel anything but competent and independent.

The isolation of new mothers at home, and from each other, along with the internalization of high expectations for competence, often keep women from speaking out about their range of emotions. They may share only half the story—the bliss they feel about their newborn—while keeping inward their stresses and anxieties, lest they be considered (or consider themselves) a "bad mother." Many experience the sense that they are failing to live up to what any mother should be able to do easily and spontaneously. Thinking that mothering is natural and therefore should come naturally, many mothers forget that it is not natural to be a mother in isolation. They may forget that in past generations, extended family and close community ties meant that women with young children had a great deal of help. And in our mothers' and grandmothers' generations, extended hospital stays after birth and visiting nurses provided some respite even if extended family were not readily available to give support.

New mothers need permission to express their emotions without judgment. Dialogues among women need to allow for the sharing of both stresses and coping strategies so that they can truly enjoy their babies without suffering a form of quiet desperation that too often leads to postpartum depression. Until women speak to each other about joys and sorrows, too many mothers will remain isolated in their experiences.

I recall a specific incident from my early childbearing days: I had recently birthed my third baby—she was perhaps 6 weeks old—and my older children were 4 and 7 years old. It was "play day" at the park for my homeschooled children, so I was trying to get us out the door for the day. I was packing lunches, the baby wanted to nurse, the older children started bickering, and suddenly I was overwhelmed and wondering what I was doing at home full time with three young children. I remember thinking, "I'm an intelligent woman. Why am I doing menial labor for no pay?" I snapped at the children, who started to cry, and then I broke down crying with them.

We eventually made it to the park; I knew I needed to be around other moms and that my kids needed a break, too. When I arrived, the other mothers cooed at the baby and praised me for being such an amazing mom with three children. This perked me up a bit—new mothers thrive on validation! Then one of the moms asked me how I was doing and I told these women that I was actually doing terribly and felt like an emotional wreck. I recounted the events of the morning. What ensued was a real communication among women—other moms started to share their struggles with their own emotions, their children, their husbands, and their choices. This was not a case of misery loves company, but rather a true opportunity for moms to be authentic and have an open dialogue. From the commiserating arose a sense of unity—we were all doing hard work and we validated each other's struggles and strengths. Nobody left that conversation feeling that she was the only one struggling to cope with multiple roles and social expectations while trying to love, enjoy, and nurture her children. What initially felt like a personal sense of being overwhelmed and incompetent was placed into a social and cultural perspective. I realized that the problem was in society's treatment of mothers, not in me.

✿ BEING A MOTHER IS SECOND NATURE, ✿ ISN'T IT?

Mothering is a combination of both learned and instinctive behaviors. Unfortunately, we are led to believe that because it is "natural" to become a mother, mothering skills will come to us naturally. Elizabeth Bing and Libby Colman clearly express the expectation most women hold for themselves as mothers: "If it is 'natural' we should be good at it" (Bing and Colman 1997). But for many women, it just isn't that simple—or that natural. As Bing and Colman write, "Instinct, self-interest and social roles don't always mesh into a perfect synergy. . . . Self sacrifice is not always a pleasure."

It is said that girls grow up learning to be mothers by emulating their own mothers and playing with dolls, just as boys become fathers through watching their dads do "man" things. It's true that traditionally girls grew up caring for younger siblings, probably making the transition to motherhood fairly smooth. Boys did not take care of other children, nor were they expected to be involved as fathers to the extent that fathers today are expected to participate in sharing the responsibility for childrearing. Years ago, women learned from other women in their community. Nowadays, much of that traditional lifestyle, as well as family and community, is lost. Perhaps more than any generation in history, young women today are isolated from the life cycles of women and the care of infants. Most women in this country give birth before they've ever changed a diaper!

Furthermore, women don't become mothers in a social vacuum. Today, the experience of motherhood is obscured by competing and conflicting social demands and expectations placed on women. For example, many women, driven by personal talents, interests and ambitions, and the desire for economic independence, among other motives, have had careers and years of childless, adult living. It is not always easy to make the transition from one role to another, especially when that requires a shift not only in daily responsibilities, but also, to some extent, in identity, and particularly when role models are not readily apparent. Many confounding issues call into question exactly what motherhood and fatherhood mean for childbearing women and for men.

Although modern parents have some things easier than ever before— washing machines and disposable diapers, for example—many factors about having a baby in modern society are highly complex. Most people don't recognize how unrealistic they are in their expectations of what it takes to care for a newborn. "It is difficult and demanding work that was never intended to be done by one adult in isolation from others" (Bing and Colman 1997). In addition, maternal love is not always an automatic response. A woman's personal life experiences may lead to an enhanced or diminished ability to feel and express love for her own child.

We must also remember not to romanticize motherhood of yesteryear. There is ample evidence that women in the past did not necessarily find motherhood entirely easy—or, for that matter, always pleasurable and romantic. For example, the use of laudanum, an opiate, as a sedative for babies was popular and widespread in the 1800s, with a notably high mortality rate. Laudanum essentially knocked babies out, giving mothers a long period of quiet while baby slept. Fortunately for today's babies and young children, this coping strategy has gone out of style.

Many of us are just not emotionally well equipped for the job due to lack of preparation. We may not have strong examples of patient, loving, gentle, creative, successful mothers, whether they have chosen to have careers or to be stay-at-home moms. We also lack experience caring for children prior to motherhood.

Living in a society that at once elevates mothers to an unrealistic and romanticized perfection while simultaneously marginalizing them so that they are economically and socially vulnerable creates many concerns that compound the difficulties in learning to be a mother. We sell family values at every turn, but do not support mothers and families: From lack of adequate maternity care leave to lack of safety in schools, mothers are vulnerable. In addition, "Our society is profoundly ambivalent about children" (Bing and Colman). Women themselves may have internalized this ambivalence and, not knowing how to express it, internalize these feelings as some kind of proof that they are bad mothers—after all, good mothers are supposed to be constantly overjoyed by motherhood, aren't they?

Many women today do not have clear maternal role models. During pregnancy, you may even find yourself thinking a lot about your own relationship to your mother, about how you were raised and perhaps pledging to do things differently or better. Your own mother (or mother-in-law) may be able to provide only limited support for your parenting choices. She may have stayed at home full time, available for her children and husband at every moment, and may therefore be unable to understand and thus even disapprove of your economic or personal need to maintain your career after becoming a mother. Conversely, your mother may have worked full time out of the home, choosing career along with family. This created its own set of problems, some of which are only now beginning to change as more women and men strive to create a better balance between work and family, increasingly integrating family awareness into the work environments. Your mother may not understand your desire to give up a career and personal opportunities to stay at home full time with your children. Your mother may take it personally when you make choices that are different from hers, feeling that you are somehow criticizing her mothering of you. This may or may not be true, yet can still lead to criticism, judgment, tension, or loss of support at a time when you need to find your own way to mother with the love and approval of your own mother, and leave you to struggle to create an identity of yourself as a mother. Women need help discovering how to connect with their own instincts while also learning about solutions and coping strategies that other mothers have developed.

Being a mother is a bit like riding a bicycle. When you start out, you need a good support person to hold on until she sees that you are steady. Then she lets go slowly and at the right time, running along beside you until you are clearly independent, steady, and confident. Eventually you're on your own. You're wobbly and probably even fall a few times. But before you know it, you are riding on your own, and your skills steadily increase until you can ride downhill, with one hand, and eventually it's "Look, Ma, no hands!" Just as with riding a bicycle, it takes time, support, patience, and practice (you'll get lots of practice!) to get the hang of mothering. But once you've been doing it for a while, you never forget how and can barely remember a time when you couldn't do it.

Women today are redefining the path of motherhood. There are many models—the stay-at-home mother; the married, full-time career woman; the single working mom; the mom who works while Dad stays at home; lesbian moms co-parenting; and adoptive moms, to name just a few. The sheer volume of moms who are raising children alone now compared to 30 years ago and the numbers of women in the workforce today have led to and now reflect an entirely changed face of motherhood in this culture.

So isn't being a mother natural? It really isn't that simple. Today women are pioneering motherhood in new ways, and have many pressures that yesterday's did not have to face. These pressures, such as deciding whether to stay at home with the baby, if this is an option, or to put your 6-week-old in childcare (and if so, what kind), affect our ability to nurture instinctively, and may interfere with what our hearts are telling us. Furthermore, women now have opportunities to be successful in professional arenas that our grandmothers just didn't have access to. Rarely did our grandmothers, when they began a family, have to question whether to leave a lucrative and stimulating job to be at home full time with no independent income and no validation of their intelligence and creativity. They did what they were expected to do, devoting their lives to their children and husbands. Many felt perfectly satisfied to do so, but others harbored feelings of frustration, depression, and lack of personal fulfillment that in turn brought resentment, sadly often internalized or unwittingly displaced on their children.

Economic pressures have a great emotional and psychological impact on modern mothers and on the ability to mother "naturally." Standards of living today require both parents to have an income. And many single moms have little choice but to have a job outside the home. Additionally, many women face issues of vulnerability and dependence if they are not contributing to the family income. These various pressures lead some mothers to shut themselves off from their instinctive, intuitive, or emotional experience of motherhood, in order to maintain the detachment that allows them to remain in the workforce without feeling too guilty.

There is also a strong sentiment in the corporate world that motherhood, emotions, and business do not mix. Although a number of women entrepreneurs have worked to change this paradigm, it is still the prevailing attitude in many professional settings. Women too often have to "turn off" their intuitive, emotional qualities for much of the day, feeling torn between their identity as mother and their professional persona. Dis-identification with our intuitive and emotional selves can lead to a diminished ability to attune and respond to the baby's needs from a natural, intuitive place. Working mothers must learn that intuition and emotional intelligence are in all settings powerful tools, not handicaps. We must empower ourselves and our women colleagues to stay intact as mothers in the professional world, and not let the corporate mentality keep us from exercising our intuitive and emotional intelligence. The world will be better for it!

Women are taught that paying too much attention to baby leads to spoiling the child. You may find that when your baby cries, your instinct is to pick the baby up and put her to your breast, but instead you hear a voice in the back of your head saying, "She nursed just 2 hours ago; you're going to spoil that child." Or perhaps it isn't a voice in the back of your head, but instead your aunt who has come to help out. So you put a pacifier in the baby's mouth, leave her in the bassinet, and eventually she falls back to sleep. This scenario repeats itself several times a day, and you assume your aunt knows best; after all, she has raised four children, and they're all doing fine. But at the next visit to the pediatrician, she tells you the baby hasn't gained enough weight and suggests supplementing breast milk with formula. Again, this goes against your intuition, but you are too worried about the baby's weight to argue. So you put the baby on a formula supplement. Nobody told you that babies who are held often gain weight faster, and that your instinct to pick up and nurse your crying baby may have prevented the need to supplement with formula. All of this, combined with the fact that you never changed a diaper before you had your baby and never even saw a woman breast feeding, sure makes mothering look anything but natural. In fact, you're starting to wish you got a Ph.D. in mothering before you started doing it!

Finally, childbirth and childrearing have become such highly medicalized experiences, with women and men relying heavily on doctors and machines to give them information on how they and their babies are doing, that mothers may not have trust in their own ability to recognize their baby's signals and needs. As in the example above, many women don't feel confident enough in their knowledge and emotional intelligence to follow their inner guidance with their babies, relying instead on the pediatrician's advice. But we must remember that it was not pediatric wisdom that led to the renewed interest in breast feeding, which has now been clearly established as the best food for baby, not just supplying excellent fuel for baby, but also promoting optimal brain development and better immunity than can bottle feeding. It was a group of intuitive and determined mothers in the Midwest who eventually formed La Leche League, the now internationally recognized breast-feeding organization. Their commitment to what they felt was best, in direct opposition to conventional medical advice, has brought about increased support for breast-feeding mothers and babies around the world.

REALISTIC EXPECTATIONS

Childbirth educators share a nearly universal quandary regarding how best to prepare women and couples for the experience of birth: How does one give parents a realistic view of birth and a useful set of skills to cope with the intensity of the experience without scaring them? If you tell parents that birth can be extremely hard and painful, and may challenge them beyond what they think are their limits, you run the risk of them either tuning you out or becoming filled with anxiety about birth. If you don't prepare them adequately for the potential (even likely) challenges of birthing, they may become extremely frightened at the intensity of the sensations of labor, and even believe something is wrong when it isn't, and they will likely blame you for not preparing them adequately.

So, too, are we challenged when trying to successfully prepare pregnant couples for the days, weeks, and months after birth. We can convey effectively neither the joys nor the stresses. The fact that the birth—which may be foremost in their minds—lies imminently in the future often prevents parents from taking in the full picture of information about the postpartum. The birth is seen as the main event, and beyond the need to gather baby supplies, it's hard to imagine life after birth. Furthermore, first-time parents often have a hard time conceptualizing that there is actually "a baby in there" enough to integrate information about new-mom and baby care. Actually having a baby in the house may seem surreal, not even concretized by the increasing volume of baby paraphernalia lying about the house or the mom's enormous belly. For most first-time parents, it is only after the baby is in arms that the reality of it sets in. Many pregnant mothers and fathers tell me during the course of prenatal visits that it is hard to believe that soon a baby will be sharing their daily lives.

For the joys of life with your newborn, you need no preparation. Each new joy is a little gift, unexpected and magical. The scent or feel of your baby's skin, the delight of looking into your husband's eyes, realizing that you are truly related through this perfect little being, the feel of your baby's hand in your own—for these, no preparation is required.

However, realistic preparation for the postpartum is essential for coping with the challenges that inevitably arise. In fact, studies demonstrate that women who have realistic expectations about the postpartum fare better as mothers than those who don't (Bing and Colman). Therefore, pregnant couples should keep an open mind about what their postpartum experience might be like, and plan for any challenges that might arise. If everything is smooth sailing, you won't need to rely on contingencies; but if you do face challenges, you will be able to meet your needs and respond well to the circumstances.

❧ THE FEMININE MYSTIQUE REVISITED ☙

Betty Friedan coined the term *feminine mystique* to describe the stereotype of the perfect, selfless superwoman. Bing and Colman suggest that the feminine mystique is still lurking in the unreasonable, even impossibly high expectations women set for themselves—especially when it comes to motherhood. We set idealized standards for ourselves that no real human could ever meet. Yet if we aren't perfect at all we do, we too often feel we are bad mothers.

Although motherhood is one of the most incredibly joyous human experiences possible, being a mother, for many women, is only one aspect of who we are. Unfortunately, the feminine mystique that women in this culture are raised with—despite the fact that more than 60 percent of all mothers work outside the home—is that mothers are expected to define themselves in relationship to their families. Yet being a mother, though incredibly satisfying, is not the entire identity of most women. We have personal interests and needs as well as talents that we want to express beyond the audience of our partners and children. Being a full-time, stay-at-home mother is increasingly rewarding. But there are also moments of tedium and boredom. Most adult women need to stimulate their minds in ways that are just not satisfied by reading

The Runaway Bunny, playing in the bathtub, and swinging at the park.

Even the most creatively involved mothers need adult engagement. And for women who have developed their talents into careers, or who dream of doing so, the life of the full-time mom might seem dreary when personal interests are entirely ignored. In fact, it is not even fair to our children to define our whole world in relation to them. To do so can put unreasonable expectations on our children to fulfill us and meet our needs. Too many mothers have been unsatisfied in their own life choices, only to try to live vicariously through their children, encouraging their kids to make the choices they in fact wanted to make for themselves—to be what they themselves wanted to be. Although I feel firmly that our children need us to be with them as much as possible, I also believe it is very important for women to be fulfilled, and to bring this richness into their relationships with their children.

As discussed earlier, many pressures come to bear on women as they become mothers. Strong social pressures to be overjoyed by motherhood leave women hesitant to express conflicting feelings. But keeping such feelings to yourself may increase your sense of social isolation and reinforce for yourself a "bad mother" image. The conflicting emotions of mothers are nearly as universal as are the joyous emotions of motherhood. Sharing these feelings among ourselves may help us recognize that it is normal to have ambivalence, and that we can find creative ways to express our full humanity. Whether you are a stay-at-home mom or a cardiac surgeon with a busy schedule, it is important for you to feel good about your choices. We must redefine what it means to be a "good mother" in terms of giving our children the very best of ourselves, as often as possible. We must also make demands on society, deconstructing the barriers that prevent us from feeling really positive about choosing to mother fully—whether these be economic, social, or emotional demands. This can happen only when we feel good about ourselves and fulfilled by our lives.

❧ SACRIFICE AND EMPOWERMENT ❧

There is no way around the fact that conscientious and committed mothering requires a significant element of personal sacrifice—whether this be in simple daily terms such as loss of sleep and quiet time for ourselves, or in bigger ways, such as sacrificing a career. For many mothers this level of devotion comes so naturally that they wouldn't dream of doing anything but surrendering their time to their baby. Even many mothers who think they will return to a job shortly after birth find themselves so attached to the baby that they decide to stay at home full time.

It can be frustrating, however, to confront the choices and make the sacrifices. Facing the loss of your career, familiar friends from work, and a social life as you move out of the fast track for the "slower" pace of motherhood, is challenging and isolating. One woman I recently spoke with had a history of fertility problems—first an inability to become pregnant, then repeated miscarriages. She finally maintained a pregnancy when she turned 40; at the same time, her career began to take off and she landed a major position in the film industry, along with a high-six-figure salary. After she had her baby, she realized she did not want to do what most mothers in the film industry do—have a daytime nanny and a nighttime nanny. She told me she didn't get pregnant to have someone else raise her baby. She cut back her hours, but doing so sabotaged her career. Today she works from home as a writer, confident she made the right choice to care for her son, and now also her daughter. Though there are financial struggles, she says she couldn't put a price tag on the precious time she has with her children while they're still young.

Women are increasingly recognizing that children require a healthy balance of quantity and quality time, and that there really are no substitutes for mommy in a child's mind. This is forcing women to rethink the feminist battle cries of the '70s and '80s and more broadly define feminism and women's empowerment to give more weight to motherhood. Many women are beginning to take pride in caring for their children full time, rather than being ashamed for making the choice to do so. Many others feel guilty if they have to or want to maintain a job or career after becoming mothers. Indeed, not all women have the opportunity to be home, and even those who are home may actually be working from home. This requires women to be masters at multitasking.

Multitasking—handling multiple roles, tasks, or responsibilities—seems to be the buzzword of this new century. Scientific evidence has revealed that mothers are more capable of multitasking than are men, even more capable than women who are not mothers. It is therefore not surprising that mothers end up doing a lot of multitasking. But no matter how engineered we are to handle it, this means a lot of juggling, which can lead to exhaustion, stress, frustration, and internal conflict. You may feel like a Jill-of-all-trades and master of none. You may feel spread thin, and that no single aspect of your life—including giving your child the attention he needs—is getting your all.

Only you can define for yourself what goals are important. However, when you make the commitment to being a mother, look beyond your own goals to the bigger picture of your baby's needs as well. It is not a small feat to integrate the two, yet it is important for you to feel good about yourself, both as a woman and as a mother. Maintaining multiple roles will provide a lot of stimulation, but can also lead to your feeling divided. You may also begin to emotionally shortchange your family as you try to cling to a piece of yourself. It is therefore important as a new mother to learn to set boundaries and priorities, and to feel good about saying no to projects and obligations that are not essential, are unsatisfying, or distract you from caring for your baby or yourself. This will prevent you from feeling so torn that you experience an identity crisis and so worn out that you feel chronically fatigued and emotionally spent.

ꙮ DEVELOPING CONFIDENCE ꙮ

It is not until a woman develops a clear sense of her own ability to be responsible for the care of a child that she begins to feel like a mother. For some women, particularly those who have already had children, this may happen fairly quickly, but for the majority of new mothers, this profound sense of confidence typically does not occur until the baby is at least 8 months old. It's amazing how the task of caring for a young baby can cause even the most competent of women to feel overwhelmed and disorganized. Many times in my practice I receive calls from women who previously had successful careers and who are now at a loss as to how to get dinner on the table while caring for a newborn. Women are often shocked at how incompetent they feel.

There are a number of factors that can undermine a woman's confidence as a mother. The support women receive from the significant people in their lives as they move through various stages and needs during pregnancy, birth, and shortly after has a tremendous bearing on psychological wellness, and thus confidence. In addition, complications during birth can reduce a woman's confidence about caring for her newborn. "Mothers who have the support of a companion during labor and delivery experience fewer complications and less postpartum depression" (Gjerdingen et al. 1991), a problem that also reduces maternal confidence. The quality of care a woman receives in the early days, weeks, and months after birth can have a significant impact on her long-term physical and emotional wellness, and on her ability to meet both her own and her baby's needs. According to Gjerdingen et al., a "review of the literature on social support and its relationship to maternal health indicates that emotional, tangible, and informational support are positively related to mothers' mental and physical health around the time of child-birth." Specifically, "mothers' postpartum mental health is related to both the emotional support and practical help (e.g., housework and child care activities) provided by the husband and others."

The hospital environment and medical and nursing staff can undermine a woman's confidence in her ability to care for her newborn. In the hospital, newborns are treated as fragile, vulnerable patients requiring constant surveillance. Thus, the mother may feel that she is anything but capable of caring for and protecting her child from the dangers in a newborn's life. If she perceives her baby to be fragile, she may not feel comfortable handling, feeding, bathing, or otherwise carrying out the normal tasks of caring for a baby.

As Sheila Kitzinger says, "Maternal emotions are urgent, raw—and often deeply disturbing." A difficult or disappointing birth experience can lead to feelings of incompetence, futility, or depression that reduce a woman's confidence as a mother. A birth that shakes your confidence can result in a sense of failure. Postpartum emotions and blurred personal boundaries can also be confusing and conflicting; thus, you lose confidence in your emotional stability and clarity. It is important to seek the help of someone who is supportive and understanding and able to help you process your difficult emotions, so you can enter motherhood with strength and confidence.

Childbearing women who receive enough support and mothering themselves are more likely to feel confident caring for their babies. At the same time, women must embrace their own sense of empowerment, and look within for the strength and confidence to mother in their own way. This is especially important for women who are making birthing or parenting decisions in opposition to the norm, or even to those of their own families of origin.

Too often, new mothers are left to their own devices to figure out how to mother when what they really need is to be mothered themselves. They need someone to prepare nourishing food, look after the other kids, run a soothing bath, look after baby while they nap, and provide comfort, guidance, and reassurance about baby care. Women need both mothering and to embrace their own role as mother. Confidence in caring for a baby is not magically born with the birth but instead develops with experience and familiarity. Parents learn over the course of the first few weeks what their baby's different sounds signify. They learn the differences among cries of discomfort, hunger, illness, and pain. With this growing knowledge comes confidence—then a cry of hunger does not inspire panic, and the cry of a colicky baby does not elicit a trip to the emergency room.

While background support around the house and encouragement with the new baby are important, meddlesome or smothering help can be detrimental. Imagine that every time a toddler learning to walk took a step or fell down someone was there telling him what he was doing wrong or holding his hand so he didn't fall—the child would likely never learn confidence in his ability to walk alone, and would never learn to help himself back up after a fall. Again, encouragement and gentle support are needed, but not overbearing advice. New parents need to learn a bit from their own trial and error to find out what works for them and their baby.

"A new mother is a target for advice—much of it conflicting," says Sheila Kitzinger. Trying to sort out your own thoughts when you feel vulnerable is a challenge. Therefore, it is best to think through as many choices as possible prior to your baby's birth, rather than trying to make decisions just after birth. For example, do research on circumcision, sleeping arrangements (crib, bassinet, family bed), breast feeding or bottle feeding, and immediate newborn tests and vaccinations prior to birth. And find one or two people—preferably women who themselves have children—whom you trust for sound experience and advice. Let them help you sort through the conflicting information you get.

A prime example is that lactation consultants often tell breast-feeding mothers and hospital nurses to feed the baby for 10 minutes at each breast during each feeding. Any mother who has breast-fed successfully, can tell you that this is unnecessary; adds to the increased stress of having to latch the baby on again, which with some newborns isn't easy; and increases nipple soreness. A mother experienced with breast feeding will tell you to relax, then feed the baby on one side fully at a nursing and on the other side at the next nursing—unless, of course, the baby is hungry enough to want both breasts in one feeding.

♌ MOTHERING ARCHETYPES ☙

As Sally Placksin tells us, in regard to postpartum care, "Many women don't realize it could and should be different"—as a culture of mothers we have "no archetypes and no paradigms." What are archetypes? They are models that embody deified human qualities. The Greek pantheon provides us with many rich archetypes and there are, of course, many gentle and tender goddess archetypes from other cultures as well—for example, the Chinese goddess Kuan Yin, mother of compassion. Kali, the Hindu goddess of fire, is one of my favorites for mothers. She is in many ways the opposite of the good-mother image—in fact, she is more often depicted as a horrible demon than anything else, a terrible specter with a necklace of skulls, hair of snakes, and a long red tongue hanging from her mouth. She reminds me of the archetypical mother protectress, never holding back on her fierceness, much as a mother would go to any lengths to protect her children. She also reminds me that we don't always have to be nice, pretty, or gentle. We just have to be real, but sometimes even fierce, to protect our own space and get our needs met.

As mothers we have the opportunity to collectively create a new paradigm, modeling how to become a mother for our daughters and other young women who look up to us. Only by demanding what we need, allowing our voices to be clear and strong, can we change social institutions significantly enough to reshape motherhood in our society. This is a challenge worth embracing, both for us and for our daughters and granddaughters. May your early days of motherhood be blessed with depth, meaning, peace, and celebration.

MODERN RITES OF PASSAGE FOR NEW MOTHERS

Prior to birth, we offer women the ceremony of a shower, at which she receives more or less helpful advice and many gifts for the new baby. When baby is born, more gifts are brought—again, for the baby. It is as if our culture says the baby is the present mom gets; why should she need anything else?

In some circles around the United States, pregnant women are treated to a MotherBlessing, also called a Blessingway, from the Dine (Navajo) term for a ceremony that takes place when a community member makes a large transition in her life (marriage, moving to another village, etc.). At a ceremony for a pregnant woman, women share positive birth stories, poems, and songs to encourage the mother and remind her of her strength to give birth. Gifts are given not only for the baby, but also for the mother—a bottle of aromatherapy oil to use at the birth, a book of poems, an IOU for a dinner brought to her house after baby is born. Her hair is brushed and she is massaged as a means of reminding her that she will be entering a new awareness as she becomes a mother.

But what rituals exist for the woman *after* she has gone through the rite of passage that is birth? There may be a baby-naming ceremony or a baptism for the family and friends to say "Welcome to the world—you are part of our community," but what is there to demarcate the woman's transition into motherhood? Where are the stories of joy and triumph, or challenge and exhaustion, as we learn to become mothers? Where is the recognition that this has been a significant life event, and has brought the mother into a new phase of her life, perhaps the most demanding she'll ever experience? Where is the establishment of a core group of support that says, "We are here for you as you work 24 hours a day, 7 days a week, to take care of this member of our family and community"?

Indeed, mothers are often overlooked at this time, and for many women the experience of motherhood is isolating and goes uncelebrated.

There are many ways, however, in which we could honor women's rite of passage into motherhood. One is to create New-Mother Blessings. This ceremony can be given by a group of women (as few as two can still constitute a group!) who agree to be the mother's support network in the early days postpartum. The mother's closest friend or female family member can take the job of New-Mother Blessing coordinator and arrange for postpartum care for the new mom. When the mother is 3 to 6 weeks postpartum, and feels more ready to take on some of her former daily routine, she can be given a ritual to mark this transition.

Of course, the ceremony doesn't mean that postpartum is over: The ceremony is merely a celebration of the mother—of her strength and accomplishment—and a renewed commitment from her community to be her support network in the coming months. This 3- to 6-week period is often a time when her friends' and family's help begins to dwindle, and people expect the mom to go back to business as usual. For others, the newness has begun to wear off. For Mom, the work is just beginning and she may feel suddenly abandoned, overwhelmed, and isolated. She has even had her last visit with her midwife or doctor, and may be feeling that things are a bit anticlimactic. This is a great time for a good celebration to honor her.

CREATING A NEW-MOTHER BLESSING CEREMONY

Decide whether this celebration will be all women or if it will include Dad and his support network also. Remember, the focus is on Mom. She might be feeling emotionally sensitive, so be thoughtful to invite people whom she feels supported by and comfortable around. Keep the gathering small enough to be intimate, cozy, and quiet, if that's the mom's mood or if baby will be asleep.

Plan the time and place, and make sure there is one person close to the mom who can help coordinate the ceremony. The mom's own house is the best place to have the New-Mother Blessing—but she should not have to do any cleaning or preparation.

Call people in advance and ask them to dress in lovely clothes. This get-together can be casual, but it should be special. Ask each participant to bring a small gift for the mother—something simple (homemade is wonderful) and something she can use on those days when she's tired, having a hard time, or just needs a reminder that she has a support network. I call these "just-for-mom presents." Ideas include a new hair clip, a lovely nursing nightgown if she is breast-feeding, a book of inspirational quotes for moms, a journal, a night of baby-sitting the older kids so she and her partner and baby can catch a movie, and a gift certificate for a massage or pedicure. Ask each guest also to bring an inspirational quote, poem, story, or song about womanhood or motherhood. If anyone plays the guitar or another instrument, all the better: Try to have some song sheets on hand so everyone can sing. Finally, each attendee should bring a potluck dish or dessert to share.

Prior to the gathering, set up a special place in the mom's house—the living room or a den works well. Place candles, flowers, and special objects that are images of motherhood (small statues, for example) and make sure there is a circle of comfortable seating. Cushions on the floor are fine. Have some massage oil on hand, as well as a towel and blanket.

For the ceremony, let your inspiration be your guide. Using the items guests have brought, create a nourishing circle to honor the mother. For example, everyone can share one thing that she loves or admires about this mom—either as a woman or as a mother. Participants can go around in a circle and share a special inspirational story from their own experience or that they've read. And each can present her gift to Mom, explaining why she selected that for her. Afterward, the mother can stretch out comfortably on the sofa to receive a foot massage from two of the guests, while everyone sings songs or continues to share stories. Mom can hold baby as she needs to, and the women gathered together can help with baby as well. Finally, the mood becomes more social, and everyone visits and enjoys a potluck.

A network like this not only serves the mother who has recently given birth, but it also bonds women who are willing to be there for each other later on, through other women's births, illnesses, and so on.

TWO

New-Mother Care around the World

*Isolation is difficult for any human, whether male or female,
but for a woman it is what psychologists call "ego dystonic," or
out of tune with our accustomed way of being. For that reason
it has the potential to be a serious stress despite the business of
our lives. We need to be mindful of the continued need to
support and be supported by one another.*

Joan Borysenko, *A Woman's Book of Life*

I've heard it said that if you wish to know about a society, notice the way it treats new mothers and babies. Looking at our society's treatment of moms and babies, I'd say we're a culture that's still in its early evolutionary stages. We are just beginning to understand the vital importance of the mother-child relationship, and we have barely begun to recognize the importance of women's experience of motherhood in shaping women's lives and the lives of their children.

As a midwife, I've had the tremendous opportunity to be with women and their families in the minutes, hours, days, weeks, and months after the births of their children. I've had a chance to observe, listen, share, and learn about what works and what doesn't. I've also had the chance to be with women from a variety of cultures as their families bathed them in the care familiar to them from their traditions. This has given me a wide-angle view of the world of postpartum care.

There is great variety in how individuals and families respond to women who have just given birth. Some families provide no support; others practically move in to help the new parents. In certain circumstances there is not enough support, sometimes there is just the right amount of help and understanding, and occasionally there is even too much involvement and interference. Friends, neighbors, employees, and colleagues may also play a helpful role—or not. Each individual woman and each family has different needs. Their relationships with extended family members, their confidence as parents, and what number child they are having, among other factors, may influence the amount of help they ask for or are offered. All of these variables come together to create a more or less supportive environment in which women become mothers.

Although we have made some progress toward recognizing the benefit of "allowing" newborns to remain with their mothers directly after birth, in our society we have made little progress toward understanding the needs of women as mothers. Many traditional cultures seem instinctively to recognize that the health of the mother is essential to the health of her newborn; thus, in the immediate postpartum period, the mother is actively attended to by her family and her village. Indeed, even many modern European countries, commonly those with the lowest infant mortality rates in the world, acknowledge the importance of the immediate postpartum period, providing women with visiting nurses at home for up to 2 weeks after birth, allowing the mother a paid maternity leave sometimes as long as 2 years, and giving the father many weeks of paid paternity leave.

Generally, in our culture, the needs of the mother are considered only in relationship to the needs of the baby—Mom needs to rest so she has energy for baby, Mom needs to drink more fluids so she has enough milk for baby. Even bonding with the baby tends to be viewed from the perspective of the baby's needs. Women who do not appear to be "bonding well" with their babies immediately after birth may be suspected by medical personnel of being potentially negligent or abusive mothers.

Little attention has been paid to the mother's needs at this time, either in relationship to herself or in relationship to how her self-image influences her ability to mother. What of a woman's need to recover her sense of herself as a woman while her identity merges with that of herself as a mother? Perhaps women need time and tending for this bonding of self with this new and enormous role. This is an area in which our culture has just begun to evolve.

In traditional societies, women could generally count on receiving a certain amount of focused postpartum care from their extended family, and at times from the greater community. It is clear that in many societies the postpartum period is one in which it is recognized that women need attention and some amount of doting. It is acknowledged that the postpartum is a sacred time when women need great protection, whether it be from evil spirits, wild animals, or "pernicious influences." The family and community work to guard, nourish, and help the mother to heal from birth, fully aware that the well-being of the child is ultimately tied to that of his mother.

Of course, not all traditional cultures should be romanticized. In some societies, postpartum-care rituals and traditions are not based on respect for women, but instead are predicated on the belief that birth is unclean or that women are weak. Therefore, women who have recently given birth are likewise considered to be unclean or feeble. Such cultures tend to be male dominated and sustain a deep disrespect for processes related to the female body. In extremes, ritual isolation practices, such as keeping the woman separate from the community for extended periods, and keeping her quite literally in the dark and in seclusion, may exist and may exert their own harmful influences.

This chapter will look at optimal traditional care of the new mother in a range of cultures, including our own contemporary society in the West, emphasizing what we can glean from such care for the nourishment of women after birth in our culture.

℀ POSTPARTUM USA: ℀
IMMEDIATELY AFTER BIRTH

Imagine that you have just given birth. Perhaps your labor was short and easy, or maybe it was long and arduous. For the first couple of hours after birth you are elated—barely able to take your eyes off your precious newborn. But after a couple of hours you're tired. Exhausted, in fact. The long night of labor catches up with you. You're ready for sleep, curled up with baby at your side. You have come through the intense journey of birth and now must embark on another—motherhood.

If you have given birth at home, and you and baby are doing well, your midwife will help you get cleaned up, perhaps in a nice herbal bath or shower, and will make sure you eat a warm meal before tucking you into bed for a well-deserved rest. Herself a woman who has likely breast-fed her children, your midwife will assist you as you learn to nurse your baby. She'll stay at your home for several hours; then, when assured that it's reasonable for her to leave, she'll go on her way knowing you're safe in the care of your support network, whether this be your partner, mother, sister, or all of them, and confident that you can reach her at a moment's notice should any questions arise.

The lights are turned down or the shades drawn, and you enter into a deep and restful sleep. When you awake several hours later, your mom or sister has another hot meal waiting for you—and food never tasted so good! You sit up in your own bed and eat, feeling like you've worked hard but are contented. Your baby wakes to nurse and you fumble around for a while trying to get it right. You're still having some difficulty so you call your midwife, who makes some simple suggestions that help you get started again. She assures you that if you continue to have trouble, she'll come back to assist you, but encourages you to relax and not worry, as anxiety only makes it harder to breast-feed easily. She also reminds you that she will be by in the morning for your first postpartum visit, and she asks how you are feeling and whether you have had some time to rest and eat. You feel reassured and go back about the business of practicing breast feeding. A new American postpartum paradigm is emerging.

Like most women in this culture, you have given birth not at home but in the hospital, and your immediate postpartum experience may not be so sublime. Chances are you have had an episiotomy—as 95 percent of women who birth in American hospitals do. The anesthetic from the suturing job to repair your perineum is wearing off and your bottom is feeling sore, so you have a giant ice pack placed against your tender perineal tissue. Nurses want to check your blood pressure every 10 minutes, you still have an IV line in your arm, and your baby has not yet been returned to your arms by the neonatal nurse, who insists the baby is not warm enough and must be kept under the radiant heat warmer across the room—or in the neonatal nursery. The obstetrician or nurse midwife left the room once the delivery was complete (placenta out, suturing done), and your husband is exhausted and emotionally overwhelmed. Staff keep walking in and out of the room to clean up, check supplies, and ready the room for the next patient immediately after you are moved to the postpartum unit. Perhaps your family is there— your mom, sister, aunt. But they, too, will leave shortly, as there is really no place for them to stay with you at the hospital.

Finally things start to quiet down. The nurse removes the IV from your arm, but the blood pressure cuff stays on for now. Staff begin to vacate your room, and your baby is brought to your side. You're hungry and it isn't yet mealtime, but you eventually receive a cold sandwich, piece of fruit, cookie, and juice in a paper bag, "specially prepared for postpartum mothers." You try to put the baby to your breast, but you're tired and unsure how to maneuver to your nipple this squirmy little package with a floppy head. You try for a while but are frustrated, thinking breast feeding was supposed to be natural, easy, and instinctive.

You are moved to a postpartum room—not nearly as spacious or as comfortably decorated as your birthing room. While you adjust to the new surroundings, you're still trying to get your baby to breast-feed. The nurse comes in and is concerned that the baby is not nursing yet. She wants to check the baby's glucose levels so he doesn't become hypoglycemic. She pricks the baby's heel for a blood sample, and goes off to find the lactation consultant. The breast-feeding specialist comes in, and is very kind and supportive, but also expresses concern that the baby nurse right away. With her help, you get the baby to latch on and suckle, and you are momentarily relieved of the anxiety that the baby might get sick because he isn't nursing enough—at only 2 hours after the birth. Satisfied that the baby is nursing, the lactation consultant leaves you, your husband, and baby alone in the room. You're exhausted, and glad to put the baby in the bassinet next to the bed or tuck him in next to you in the hospital bed, and finally you fall asleep. In 2 hours nurses wake you and the baby to monitor both of your temperatures, check your blood pressure, evaluate your bleeding, and recheck the baby's glucose levels. The latter leaves you with a lingering anxiety that the baby is not able to get enough nourishment from your breast, but fortunately the blood test comes back normal.

After a day or two of this, if there are no problems, the pediatrician will come in and sign a release for the baby to be discharged from the hospital. Finally, you'll head home, relieved to be going to a familiar place and excited to bring your baby out into the world.

The postpartum scenario will be slightly different for the 25 percent of women who have had cesareans. Most are not able to hold their babies for the first couple of hours after birth, as they are now under postoperative care. Many will find that breast feeding with an abdominal incision entails some challenging moments—they'll find it uncomfortable and awkward to maneuver the baby. They may require pain medication for the first couple of days, which also reaches the breast-feeding baby, and the care of the incision requires additional attention. Although all women require rest after birth, women who have had cesareans may find it more difficult to handle stairs, lift the baby, or meet their own basic needs. Furthermore, they may be assimilating the events of a difficult birth. For some women having a C-section is easily accepted emotionally, but for others there are varying levels of disappointment, anger, or feelings of failure.

When you arrive at home, perhaps you find that your mom or a friend or another relative has been there and brought food for you and maybe even tidied up for your arrival. Often, however, the new parents arrive home only to be the host to friends and family who have come to see the baby. Mom feels she needs to look presentable, have food for guests, and make her home clean. Rather than resting and being doted on, many a new mom ends up being hostess in the days after birth while all attention is given to her little one. It's no wonder that postpartum depression, as we'll see in chapter 5, is prevalent in our society.

⟋⟋ IMMEDIATELY AFTER BIRTH: ⟋⟋ A GLIMPSE AT TRADITIONS

Judith Goldsmith, in her classic book *Childbirth Wisdom*, illustrates with the following images the type of care that many women in West African societies receive in their villages in the days after the birth of the baby:

> Engwala's mother was dancing in the courtyard of her house. She sang to women around her . . . and to all the neighboring houses, of the new day ahead and the new child in the family.
>
> Inside, Engwala rested by the fire, wrapped up well, her baby asleep in the folds of her blanket. She was sleepy but could not take her eyes from the new little one.
>
> Occasionally one of her sisters would come to check on her, but for the most part she sat quietly, listening to the women celebrating outside.
>
> Engwala's mother and sisters came back to sit with her. Inside it was still dark. They rested and talked until the day grew warm. Engwala's mother massaged her abdomen well. . . .

Eventually Engwala is led to a stream, where with other women she relaxes in the cool water, leaning back with her legs open and her eyes closed. Her older sister holds the baby. The new mother rests awhile after the other women get out of the water, then she joins the women to help with the afternoon chores.

In many West African tribes—and in other places around the world—women continue to receive such healing massage and care daily, sometimes interspersed with resuming their daily tasks, but equally as often in lieu of social responsibilities for as long as the first 40 days after birth.

Such care is common throughout the world; various similar traditions are substituted in different cultures. Indeed, I have witnessed such care from German mothers, Puerto Rican mothers, South African mothers, and Ecuadoran mothers alike, when coming to visit their daughters who have given birth here in the United States. One thing is consistent: Women could expect to be cared for after the birth. Certainly a woman does not need to be in a hut in West Africa to receive nourishing postpartum attention. This is contrary to the experience of most women in the West, where few cultural models exist to ensure that we are cared for during this time. As Sally Placksin writes about her own postpartum and her research into other women's experiences of their postpartum care, ". . . nothing went into action automatically. If a postpartum plan or supportive network existed, it was . . . the mother's responsibility to start from scratch and put it all together" (Placksin 2000).

❧ LYING-IN ☙

The time after birth, which is reserved for the mother to rest and recuperate, is referred to as the *lying-in* time. In my midwifery practice I typically see American women receiving help from their own mothers for about 5 days after the birth. During this time the grandmother cooks, helps with the housework, and often takes care of the baby so Mom can get some rest. The new dad will often also take off several days to a week from work to help around the house and get to know the new little one. Then, generally, Grandma goes home and Dad goes back to work, leaving the new mom to care for herself and the baby. Sometimes the dad will work while the grandmother visits, and then can take off the next week, giving the new mom 2 weeks to adjust.

When I work with women from other countries of origin, I typically see their mothers coming for a lengthier stay—sometimes because they have traveled from abroad, but also because extended postpartum care is part of their cultural tradition. In such instances, it is not uncommon for the new grandmother to stay 4 to 6 weeks after the birth, providing the mother with traditional food, and also helping around the house. Because breast feeding is more common in many other countries, women who come from Europe, Central and South America, and Africa are more likely to receive constructive help with breast feeding from their female relatives than are those whose mothers are from the United States. Most moms here were bottle-fed, as were their mothers, and therefore have little experience with breast feeding.

Thus the older generation may be able to offer little or no assistance in this area, and may at times, as discussed in chapter 3, actually be a hindrance to establishing a successful breast-feeding relationship.

It wasn't long ago that there was a rich tradition of lying-in the United States. Wertz and Wertz, in their well-researched book *Lying In: A History of Childbirth in America*, discuss this practice in detail. For example, to the New England colonists, the birth of a baby presented the opportunity for a social event: "Childbirth was a woman's event and the woman invited the help of friends and neighbors, and the entire community would pitch in, not only to help with the birth, but to help with the postpartum care. Anywhere from 6 to 8 weeks was considered a suitable lying-in period, during which a woman rested, and other people helped for free with the care of her other children and the house. . . . At the end of the period it was custom for the woman to give a party . . . she would invite all of the women who had helped during the birth and lying-in period, and they would have really a women's festival, and there's been nothing like it ever since." (Wertz and Wertz 1977).

It wasn't until the 1920s that there was an en masse movement toward childbirth in the hospital. At this time, there was also a trend away from women wanting their own mothers to care for them after birth (Placksin 51). It was considered de rigeur and proper to have professional nursing care for the baby, and those who could afford to do so did. Frequently, women stayed in hotel-like rooms in the hospital for up to 2 weeks after the birth. Popular advertisements of the day convinced women that the hospital environment was a safer one for newborns than was home, where babies could be exposed to life-threatening germs. Middle- and upper-class women relished the hospital stay, and supported a trend of moving mother-care away from the home and family.

With the advent of World War II, hospitals became less luxurious, turning into the "more efficient delivery machines we recognize today" (Placksin 2000). Today high prices in obstetrics have led to consumer demand for better services—thus the resurrection of the "luxury hotel" environment of labor and delivery rooms in many large hospitals. But the lack of attention given to postpartum is evident in the lack of attention that has been given to hospital postpartum units.

In cultures worldwide and as diverse as the Huichol of Mexico and the Mbuti of Africa, recovery time varied significantly and may have been as short as several hours—in this case, the woman went back to her social duties shortly after birth—or it might have been as long as 3 months before a woman was expected to resume her full responsibilities. It was typical for women to be given special postpartum treatments for 2 weeks after the birth, and many societies considered 40 days to be a sort of magic number, after which the mother could safely reenter into the daily workings of her society.

Interestingly, in many cultures it was thought best for a woman not to rest too long after birth, and that actually resuming some amount of activity was healthiest for her recovery. The Modoc of California were purported to believe that "a woman who arose soon had an easier time in the birth of her subsequent child" (Goldsmith 1984). Women generally took several days of rest in bed, an additional 1 to 4 weeks of rest, performing only household responsibilities, and then rejoined their community work. Furthermore, cross-culturally it was important that women rest in certain positions. Upright or semi-reclining positions were considered optimal for facilitating the expulsion of blood from the uterus and helping the uterus to regain its pre-pregnant size. It is true that when women lie down after birth, the afterbirth blood tends to pool and clot in the uterus and upper vaginal canal. When this clotting is significant, it can prevent the uterus from contracting efficiently and may cause excessive bleeding.

Occasionally, we find historical references to tribes in which the women took no rest after birth. Anthropologist Margaret Mead, reporting on birth in a Samoan village, noted that women gave birth, visitors came to see the new baby, and, when they left, the mother resumed her daily activities. Similarly, among tribes in the Congo and in Argentina, anthropologists have noted that there is no rest for women who have just given birth—they simply return to work immediately (Goldsmith). However, although stories of women giving birth in the fields and immediately resuming work are the stereotypical accounts of "native birth," it is clear that allowing the mother a period of rest with her baby was the more widely practiced postpartum custom.

Many researchers have been tempted to attribute postpartum mother-rest customs to issues of "ritual pollution" of the mother, but evidence exists that "the mother's rest after childbirth was not of a ritual nature . . . its length might be adjusted according to the condition of the new mother" (Goldsmith). Such events as the mother's milk coming in and the baby's cord falling off might have represented milestones from which the length of appropriate postpartum rest was judged.

Indeed, in most cultures in which postpartum practices have been studied, it is evident that the mother is not ritually separated from others, but that her family and community actively support and visit her regularly. Birth in most societies is a social event, drawing in the extended family and close friends to tend to the needs of the mother, as she tends to the needs of her baby.

Although the length of recovery time in traditional cultures may vary, postpartum practices have strikingly similar themes. The modes of care delivery may also differ, but the similarities are great enough that we may want to explore the significance of some of these practices and look at how they could be adapted for us.

⸾⸎   RITES OF PASSAGE   ⸎⸽

In the story of Engwala, the women of her family are celebrating a momentous occasion, and they are alerting the whole village to the fact that a joyous event has occurred. So, too, in our culture do we celebrate the birth of a baby as an important occasion. We attach balloons to the mailbox, put bows on the front door, and receive gifts for the newborn—booties, picture frames, gift certificates to baby stores. The mother and father alike are congratulated. But what attention is really given to the mother and her specific physical, emotional, mental, and spiritual needs? Rituals and traditions are frequently more significant in nature than just celebration. Rituals serve as rites of passage—events with psychological significance to the initiate that extend beyond the mundane. Rites of passage generally symbolize the change from one status to another. They usher societal members into a new peer group through initiation ceremonies.

To the Gbandes people of Liberia, the Maikal Hills people of India, and the Aztecs of Mexico, childbirth was considered a battle the mother waged. The Maikal Hills people say, "A man fights in the open air with sword and spear; a woman's battle is in the dark behind shut doors" (Goldsmith). Among the Comanche, women who died in childbirth were given honorary funerals, ceremonies equivalent to those accorded to men who had died in battle. And today among the Lakota peoples and others who participate in the Sundance Ceremony, which entails enduring a painful impaling of the chest with spiked pegs, women are exempt, as childbirth is considered an equivalent if not greater spiritual and endurance challenge. After childbirth, in such cultures, women are treated as honored members of the tribe. A woman might emerge from her birthing hut after her lying-in period with a red string around her waist and be led proudly by the village chief or priest around the village for all to see that she has taken her place as a mother in the community.

Social customs surrounding childbirth have served to initiate mothers into their new status as mothers, at the same time welcoming them into the inner sanctum of motherhood. Rites of passage into motherhood that symbolically, emotionally, and physically demarcate the passage into motherhood may ease a new mother's sense of isolation and anxiety, as mothers share with each other not only their joys, but their struggles as well.

❧ POSTPARTUM FAMILY SUPPORT ☙

According to Sally Placksin in the useful book *Mothering the New Mother,* most women don't get the kind of postpartum care they really need. Some women realize that the problem is a deficit in society, not in themselves; but, unfortunately, they still don't get the care they need unless they line it up themselves. This is in stark contrast to postpartum cultures worldwide where the new mother is doted on, tended to, massaged, and cared for until she is ready to emerge into her larger cultural group, now a rested mother.

After birth in this country, frequently the mother's mother will come and help her daughter. However, mother-daughter relationships are not always without tension, and the new grandmother may have very definite ideas about new-baby care in contrast to the mother's own. Generational ideas of postpartum mother and baby care are often quite different. Many women, for example, want to breast-feed their babies, but find that their own mothers not only lack experience in this area but also discourage their efforts. Breast-feeding babies usually want to nurse more often than do formula-fed babies, because breast milk digests faster than formula. Many grandmothers believe the baby wants to nurse so often because she isn't getting enough to eat from the breast. This can be terribly anxiety-provoking to a new mother who has not yet successfully breast-fed a child and learned about nursing patterns.

Even when mother-daughter relationships are excellent, many grandmothers want to tend to the baby so Mom can rest, rather than take charge of all the other household responsibilities so Mom can care for the baby herself and rest along with baby. This can also be disruptive to the mother-baby relationship.

Finally, even under the best of circumstances, people today are living busy, fast-paced lives that make time out for new mom and baby care difficult to fit in. Families may live a great distance from each other, making postpartum care of the mother less likely due to time constraints and the expense involved in travel. Sisters and friends may have families of their own, making it hard for them to get away. A helpful grandmother may be able to put in only a week of postpartum visiting time, and other family members and friends perhaps can't help at all. This puts an enormous amount of pressure on the new mother to care for herself and to get back "into the swing of things" more quickly than she might be physically or emotionally prepared to do. It also puts tremendous pressure on the new dad, who may not be allowed much time off from work to care for his family. Frequently, he is torn between work and home, cutting corners where he can at work to leave early, or working a full day and coming home exhausted at night to be greeted by a possibly drained and emotional new mom or older siblings needing to be bathed, tucked in bed, and have stories read. Then there is the laundry. . . .

In the United States, new babies are the center of attention. Mom is expected to look the part of the made-up and happy mother. Women themselves perpetuate this every time they dress up for company. I'm astounded at the number of times I've returned for a 1- or 3-day postpartum visit to find the new mom dressed and made up, entertaining company. It is important for a mother to be able to show off her accomplishment and share her joy and pride, but it is equally important that she rest, recuperate, and honor the sacredness of the postnatal period.

In a traditional society, postpartum visitors tend to the needs of the new mother; they don't expect her to entertain them. According to Goldsmith, for example, "In Fiji, two girls from the mother's side, two from the father's, and both grandmothers tended the mother until the tenth day, when the husband took over." In fact, in many societies women return to their own mother's house to give birth, and thus are tended to after the birth for a period of time. A woman recently told me that in her husband's Greek family, the grandmother of the new baby will come sleep in the bed with her daughter (or daughter-in-law) and the baby, while the husband is relegated to sleeping in another room. Grandmother is there to assist when the baby wakes in the night, and to tend to any needs the mother may have.

In Ethiopia, a new mother can expect the company of older women in the village, and among the Cherokee postpartum care of the mother also receives detailed attention. My friend, herbalist and Cherokee elder David Winston, shares the following: "In the Cherokee tradition women, after giving birth spend a time of 28 days in relative seclusion. During this time they do not go to ceremonies, cook, or care for children or husbands. They are cared for. Usually, the grandmothers, aunts, or sisters provide them with food and all of their other needs. The room or rooms the woman stays in are kept comfortably warm and slightly dark to make it easier for the baby. The mother and baby spend most of their time talking, sleeping, and creating a strong bond. The woman's diet is very specific with lots of blood-nourishing foods such as deer liver, red berries, green leafy vegetables if available, lots of soups or broths, and easily digestible foods such as chestnuts and hominy corn. Herb teas are also given to help prevent infection, prevent colic, and to nourish the mother and child. After 28 days there is a ceremony for the woman and she and the baby rejoin the greater society."

Winston adds that with "relative seclusion," the mother decides how much contact she wants, no one else, reminding us that these were not customs created to oppress women. "Cherokee people are matriarchal," Winston says, "and the women's ceremonies were created by spirit as revealed to women."

❧ HEAT AND HEALING ☙

If any single theme from traditional postpartum care emerges from one culture to the next worldwide, it is the importance of keeping the new mother warm. In fact, heat usually goes beyond just keeping the ambient temperature warm, but also incorporates techniques for infusing heat deeply into the woman's body specifically for the purpose of facilitating postpartum healing. Techniques include the use of heated stones, leaves, herbs, sand, and oil applied to the mother's abdomen, or even her entire body. Western direct-entry midwives have adopted the term *mother roasting,* coined from the Southeast Asian postpartum heat practices referred to as such.

Mother roasting and other practices of "fire-rest," as they are called by midwife and acupuncturist Raven Lang (Lang 1987), have many benefits. They reduce the uterine cramping that often occurs after birth, promote rest and relaxation, and help to discharge excess fluid that has accumulated during the pregnancy (which many women sweat out in the days, and especially nights, after birth, only to find themselves chilled from sweating). Mother roasting is thought to reduce postpartum uterine bleeding and discharge, and to help restore the organs to their nonpregnant tone and size. According to Lang, fire treatments were practiced throughout Southeast Asia, including the Philippines, Malaysia, Sumatra, Sarawak, Thailand, Vietnam, and Borneo. Cultures from Australia to Arizona also practiced mother-roasting techniques.

In Southeast Asia, the practice of mother roasting consists of having the mother lie on a wooden bed, underneath which a fire is lit and kept burning.

> During the pregnancy, the father of the coming baby chopped and split wood for the Mother Roasting in a sacred manner. The wood was stacked in a special way and would not be used under any circumstances prior to the birth of the baby. Once the baby was born, the house was literally shut down; doors and windows were closed. . . . When the postpartum house was closed down, a sign was put on the door telling the community that the birth had been completed and who has been born. This helped to keep the greater community away and to serve important aspects of postpartum concerns: The air could be contained, the temperature maintained, and there would be less disturbance of rest and sleeping. The father's important task then began, and continued non-stop for the duration of the lying-in period. He would light a fire in a sacred manner under or beside the bed of the postpartum duo. In some instances the fire was quite large and the intent was to keep it that way. If the fire became too strong, the woman dipped a piece of cloth into a pot of water to extinguish part of the fire; but for the most part she tried to stay as warm as possible (Lang 1987).

In some cultures, such as in Thailand, the mother would simply lie close to the fire and rotate her body day and night. In Vietnam, the fire was kept lit under the bed for 1 month after the birth, a typical length of time for fire treatments in Southeast Asia. Sometimes heated bricks wrapped in warm blankets were used as a substitute for a fire. In the Philippines, new mothers would sit on a low chair with a slatted bottom. Under the chair was placed a glowing bowl of coals, and over the mother were placed blankets to create a tent. They were to remain in this heat until a sweat was generated (Lang 1987).

Warm sand and ash treatments were also common. In one Australian culture, among the Tiwi, a fire is lit at the onset of labor. After birth, the fire is extinguished and the mother squats over the warm ashes. Some of the warm ashes are also wrapped in a cloth that is then held against her abdomen.

Many Native American nations, including the Hopi, Zuni, San Carlos, and Cahuilla, practiced heat treatments using warmed sand. Herbalist and acupuncturist Roy Upton shared the following Cahuilla tradition with me: After birth, a grandfather or uncle would dig a shallow pit and stoke a fire in it all day to heat the ground. At sunset he raked out the coals, covered the ground with pine boughs and blankets, lay the new mother in it, covered her with blankets and then sand up to her breasts so she could still nurse, and gave her chaparral tea to drink. Then he told her stories and sang to her. The next day they would dig her out, clear out the pit, start the fire, and begin again. This was done for 7 days.

Judith Goldsmith reports that the warm sand bed is also used in Australia, and that the practice may have been brought there by an ancient wave of migration from China. This indicates that the warm sand bed practice is ancient, perhaps one of the oldest forms of postpartum heat treatments. According to Lang, the purpose of such rituals is to get the breast milk flowing easily, firm the uterus, reduce cramps, and help reduce bleeding. Certainly these practices are comforting, and allow the mother to sleep when needed, do nothing but care for her baby, and enjoy peace and quiet at her leisure before recommencing her social responsibilities.

LAKOTA LORE

After birth in the Lakota tradition, the parents would seek the services of a *Heyoka* in order to choose a name. Two beaded pouches would be made. One in the shape of a turtle and the other a lizard. The umbilical cord would be placed in one of them with sweetgrass and sage placed in the other. This way potentially bad spirits could not find the umbilical cord.

—Roy Upton, Herbalist

Many anthropologists interpret the postpartum practices of traditional cultures as ritualistic methods of purifying unclean women after birth. Sometimes this may have been the case, but, in fact, most often these practices were likely done to support the mother in her transition and give her time to rest and bond with her baby (Lang 1987). When looking at birth from an anthropological perspective, it seems that women in traditional societies commonly not only had relatively easy births, but also enjoyed rapid and complete recoveries with minimal complications, especially in regard to postpartum blood loss. Also, rarely were there problems with breast-milk production (Lang 1987).

According to traditional Chinese medicine, heat is highly significant for the woman who has recently given birth. One of the three major factors considered important for the health of postpartum women is "sparing the exterior." According to traditional Chinese herbalist Andy Ellis, this means protecting against wind and avoiding cold drafts. Childbirth is thought to deplete what in Chinese is called the *wei chi*. The wei chi is the body's protective immune capacity, found specifically on the surface of the body and in the lungs. Special herbs protect the woman and nourish the wei chi, and the woman is expected to remain indoors for 1 month after birth.

MOXABUSTION FOR ESSENTIAL POSTPARTUM CARE

Midwife Raven Lang wanted to find a way to provide her clients with the type of "mother roasting" that her research on postpartum care revealed was routine for women in Southeast Asia. Combining her knowledge as a practitioner of traditional Chinese medicine (TCM) with her experience as a midwife, she realized that fire is an element essential in TCM for restoring balance after birth. She then looked for TCM models of care that might apply to mothers in the West.

Although I believe the body has an intrinsic ability to restore balance after birth if nutrition and lifestyle have been healthy during the pregnancy, many women nonetheless love the warmth and soothing feeling of a moxabustion treatment.

In TCM, there is an area of the body known as the *Ming Men*, meaning "Life Gate," or "Life Gate Fire." This correlates to the TCM concept of the kidneys, which are said to govern the functions of reproduction, sexuality, growth, and decline. It also controls the relaxation of the pelvis, which allows the baby to be born. According to herbalist, acupuncturist, and midwife Valerie Appleton, "The Ming Men, being a 'gate,' opens and closes. To give birth, the Ming Men must open, and proper recovery necessitates closure of the Ming Men." Cesarean delivery also causes the Ming Men to open. Rest and heat are the two cardinal factors that facilitate proper closure of the Life Gate.

According to Lang (1987), incomplete recovery can lead to chronic health problems and general weakness, which may become worse with each successive birth. Heat treatments, in the form of moxabustion, may be added to the postpartum-care routine to ensure optimal recovery. They may be done by a midwife, a relative or friend, or even the mother herself.

Moxa is an herb called Chinese mugwort (*artemesia argyi*), traditionally used internally for the treatment of gynecologic problems. For external use it comes in the form of a rolled stick, much like a cigar, but completely covered by a fine linen paper. The end of this stick, when lit and held close to the skin, sends a deep, penetrating warmth into the area. The technique of moxabustion was featured in an article in the *Journal of the American Medical Association* (November 11, 1998), in which researchers concluded that the technique is reliable for turning babies from the breech to the head-down position. No research has yet been published on its use for postpartum care, but midwives who incorporate this technique into their clinical practices, and mothers who have received this technique, can attest to its value.

TO GIVE A MOXABUSTION TREATMENT

Caution: Use fire safety precautions when treating with moxa.

1. Have the mother lie in a comfortable position on her side or belly. Use pillows to support her if her breasts are sore or enlarged from breast feeding. Make sure the room is warm.

2. Provide some ventilation, but do not allow the mother to receive a chill or draft. A window may be slightly open on the opposite side of the room, or use "little smoke" moxa in cold weather. It is more difficult to light, but does not emit as much smoke.

3. Peel the outer paper wrapper off the moxa stick. Light the moxa stick with the inner paper left on it. Blow on the end until it is a burning ember. Roll off any excess ash in an ashtray or dish until the tip of the moxa becomes slightly cone-shaped.

4. The area on the body you want to treat extends over the sacrum on the back and on the front just above the pubic bone to about an inch below the navel to 3 inches on either side of the midline of the lower abdomen.

5. Holding the moxa stick 1–2 inches over the correct area, begin to move the stick in tiny circles about 2 inches in diameter, until the area becomes warm and slightly pink. Then move to an adjacent spot until the whole area has been treated. Do not touch the mother with the moxa, and periodically knock off ashes into the ashtray or dish to prevent them from falling on her. Do not treat to the point of burning or stinging pain, and instruct the mother to tell you if any area is becoming too hot.

6. Continue treating the back for 15 minutes, then "massage the heat inward" for several minutes before proceeding to treat the abdomen.

7. A woman may give herself a moxa treatment on the abdomen if no one is available to do the treatment on her back.

> 8. To extinguish the moxa, place it upside down into a small dish of sand, run the tip under water until it is no longer lit, or use a specially made moxa extinguisher.
>
> 9. Begin treatments the first day after birth, and continue daily for 1 to 2 weeks.
>
> *Note:* See Resources for information on obtaining moxabustion products.

If you choose not to use moxabustion, but want to practice some form of fire-rest for the mother, a simple way is just to keep the mother very warm in the early postpartum days. Keeping the temperature in the house or apartment warm is the easiest way to do this. Ensure that neither Mom nor baby gets dehydrated by giving plenty of fluids to the mom and allowing the baby to breast-feed freely.

✼   MASGE   ✼

Massage can help postnatal aches and cramps pass much more quickly, thus relieving muscular tension that developed during the hard work of labor and easing afterbirth uterine cramps. A postpartum massage can also soothe the muscles, joints, and tissue that stretched to accommodate your growing baby.

According to writer Carroll Dunham, in her book *Mamatoto: A Celebration of Birth,* women all around the world have had massages after their babies were born. Malaysian women received daily abdominal massage from specially trained masseuses, while women in Europe and North American had kneading treatments that were popular until the 20th century. From as far east as the Maikal Hills in India to the Jicarillo people of Mexico in the West, women had their bodies rubbed with lotions made from herbs and warm oils. Mayan women received 20 postpartum massages! In most cultures, emphasis was on abdominal massage for rubbing the womb back into both size and shape, but also into its proper place in the pelvis.

In Ayurvedic medicine, a several-thousand-year-old system of traditional medicine from India and now practiced worldwide, postpartum women, as a routine, are given massage, different types of baths, and diets medicated with herbs that are nourishing and revitalizing to the mother (Bhagwan Dash, *Embryology and Maternity in Ayurveda.* New Delhi: Delhi Diary, 1975).

Massage also has a place in the postpartum medical care of women in contemporary China. At the Shanghai Nanshi Maternity and Infant Health

Hospital, traditional Chinese doctors make use of herbal remedies, acupuncture, and massage "to regulate the balancing tendency of the dynamic body to . . . recover the normal homeostate of the body" (Shi Py 1995).

Although a professional massage from someone who knows about the changes of a postpartum woman's body is a wonderful gift, a person does not have to be a professional massage therapist to give a good massage. Humans thrive on loving touch, and such touch—combined with common sense, a bit of intuitive awareness, and a willingness to ask the mom what feels good—will relieve the aches of many a postpartum mom.

POSTPARTUM MASSAGE: A HOW-TO

Set up the mom in a comfortable, warm place, such as on her bed or on a soft carpeted floor. Place an old sheet under her to protect the furnishings if you are giving a massage with oil. Make sure there are no drafts in the room, so she doesn't become chilled. Arrange enough time for a thorough massage, as well as time for the new mom to rest for a while afterward. A 30–60-minute massage followed by a 30-minute rest is perfect.

The mother should try to wear minimal clothing: a pair of panties and perhaps a camisole, or no shirt at all. Drape another sheet over her if she is modest, and to keep warm the exposed areas that you are not working on. If a breast-feeding mother is going to lie on her belly, she may need some pillows placed strategically under her to keep her breasts lifted off the mattress or floor. This will prevent her breasts from becoming sore and compressed. Have handy any massage oil you intend to use.

With a small amount of oil, begin by massaging the feet, using slow, steady strokes and slight downward pressure. Ask the mom if your touch is too light or too firm. Using her occasional feedback, you'll learn what feels good to her and what doesn't, modifying your techniques as you go along.

Progress up the legs, kneading out any kinks you feel under your hands. When you get to the area of the buttocks and hips, keep in mind that she might be a bit tender, especially if she's had her back rubbed a lot during the labor. Deep, downward and inward pressure often feels healing after giving birth—as if everything is being pressed back into its proper place.

Gentle pressure and kneading will also feel good as you work your way up the back, shoulders, and neck. Finish by massaging the head, then work your way slightly down the back again. Giving birth causes most women to exert their neck, shoulder, and back muscles. Mom will probably appreciate a little extra attention in these areas. A penetrating postpartum massage lasts for a minimum of 30 minutes.

When you have completed the massage, cover her with the sheet and let her rest and soak in the relaxation for a while.

Ideally, postpartum massage is given to the new mother daily for at least 1 week after birth, beginning about 24 hours after the baby was born.

MASSAGE OILS FOR THE NEW MOM

There are many wonderful massage oils and aromatherapy products on the market. It's also easy to prepare your own special blend for after the baby is born. A massage oil is a great gift for a new mom—especially when accompanied by the promise of a massage after the birth!

To prepare your own massage oil, all you need are three items:

1. A plastic squeeze bottle for dispensing and storing the oil

2. A base or carrier oil, a mild oil that comprises the main body of the oil in the blend

3. The scent oil or oils (favorites for deep relaxation include sandalwood-vanilla blend, lavender, rose geranium, and jasmine)

Purchase a plastic squeeze bottle from a pharmacy, or see Resources. A 4-ounce size bottle is fine. The carrier oil constitutes the main volume of oil. Almond oil is my favorite, as it is light, has very little scent, absorbs easily, and is relatively affordable. Grapeseed oil is another favorite of many massage oil companies; apricot kernel and avocado oils are used as well. Use any of these alone or in combination.

As for scents, you'll want a good-quality essential oil or a combination of several scents. These are available at large natural food stores, aromatherapy shops, and through mail-order companies (see Resources). Essential oils are highly concentrated substances and are *for external use only*. It takes only a small amount of essential oil to scent a 4-ounce bottle of almond oil.

To prepare, fill your 4-ounce bottle nearly to the top with the almond oil and add 20–40 drops of any single essential oil or a combination of scents. Shake well. Some herbalists add 1 teaspoon of vitamin E to prolong the shelf life of the almond oil. As an antioxidant, it prevents oils from becoming rancid.

Suggested scents for new moms include sandalwood and vanilla in combination, jasmine, amber, lavender, rose geranium, and clary sage. Each of these oils has its unique qualities, but all are useful for preventing and reducing depression, mental anxiety, and stress-related fatigue. In addition, oils such as jasmine and clary sage have been used to reduce uterine cramping, and can be applied, in the diluted form in the massage oil, to the abdomen.

Store the massage oil away from heat and direct sunlight.

If you are interested in learning more about aromatherapy, I recommend *Aromatherapy: A Complete Guide to the Healing Art*, by Kathi Keville and Mindy Green (see Bibliography).

Postpartum positioning of the uterus is given no attention in Western medical tradition—and not even much attention by midwives in the United States and most European countries. However, it was commonplace in various traditional cultures throughout the world to "massage the uterus back into place." Goldsmith notes that abdominal massage for such purposes was practiced in the Philippines, where it was said to "return the womb to its normal position," and all the way to the west coast of Africa, where after the birth the midwife "placed her head low on the mother's abdomen and pressed upward with it to bring the womb back into place."

Herbalist Rosita Arvigo, in her book *Sastun: My Apprenticeship with a Maya Healer,* describes the importance of massage to ensure proper uterine placement, as learned from her mentor, traditional healer Don Elijio. Don Elijio told Arvigo, "The womb is the woman's center. . . . If her uterus is not sitting where it should be, nothing is right for her; she will have late periods, early periods, clotted blood, dark blood, painful periods, yeast infections, no babies, weakness, headaches, backaches, nervousness, and all manner of ailments." He went on to tell his student that many women have a displaced uterus due to, among other things, high heels: "Modern life, carrying heavy loads too soon after child. . . . Midwives, doctors, and nurses who don't put belly band on the woman after delivery to ensure the uterus is returned to its rightful place." Tension, stress, and anxiety further weaken uterine muscles, according to Don Elijio.

Although it may be hard to find many practitioners who are able to do this for you postpartum, if you are interested in traditional uterine replacement techniques, a skilled midwife should be able to help you determine whether your uterus is in its proper place or if it has become tipped to one side or the other. And Rosita Arvigo herself teaches the traditional uterine massage techniques in workshops around the country. In general, however, women who are in good shape before the birth, push easily and naturally during the birth of the baby, and have adequate rest afterward, will naturally regain proper uterine placement. Chapter 7 describes gentle yoga exercises that also promote proper uterine placement and good pelvic-floor and abdominal tone.

✂ WRAPPING THE BELLY ✂

Don Elijio's recommendation was not just for uterine massage but, as mentioned above, also to place a "belly band on the woman after delivery to ensure the uterus is returned to its rightful place." Again, this practice is not unique to Don Elijio or the Mayan people, but has been noted worldwide as a traditional postpartum practice. According to Goldsmith, "The abdomen was bound to ensure the complete drainage of blood, as well as to help contract the uterus." In *Embryology and Maternity in Ayurveda*, it is advised that the mother's abdomen be massaged with an herbally medicated oil, then a large piece of white cloth should be wrapped tightly around her abdomen. It is believed to prevent *vata*, or wind, from accumulating in the abdomen, which is thought to be injurious to the new mother.

Indeed, in the first month postpartum the uterus returns to its prepregnant size. Many postpartum practices are intended to facilitate this process. The belly-wrapping procedure is thought to prevent excessive postpartum bleeding while maintaining the uterus in a contracted position—which would, in fact, do just this. It also maintains warmth in the area of the Ming Men (see page 48).

Various materials were effective for abdominal binding, including a long strip of cloth, leather, bark cloth, and braided grass or vegetable fibers. If the material used for binding was coarse, a soft pad may have been placed under it to cover the abdomen. Materials were of various thickness, ranging from a thin rope to a band of fabric a foot wide (Goldsmith 1984). The band may have been worn for several days or for up to 3 months, sometimes being tightened a bit each day as the abdomen decreased in size. It should not, however, have been wrapped too tight. In some tribes, a wearing such a belt around the belly was in itself a symbol of motherhood.

Belly binding is an easy practice for modern women to adopt, and for many women the feeling of the belly wrap is comforting. Use a long strip of fabric, 8 to 10 inches wide, and approximately 5 feet in length. Thin cotton is ideal. To wrap your belly, place one end of the fabric midline on your abdomen, extending from just above the pubic bone (your pubic hair line) to just under the navel. Begin wrapping the fabric, sashlike, around your belly, keeping within this line, just below your waist, until you come to the other end of the fabric, wrapping firmly but not too tightly (you should be able to fit one finger between your skin and the fabric). Use safety pins (or diaper pins) to fasten down the end. Wear this for as much of the day as you please. Some women prefer to remove the belly wrap while they sleep. Having your partner or postpartum support person help you put on the wrap will make it easier to get just the right tightness. Continue to use the belly wrap for up to 2 weeks after the birth.

❧   HERBS   ☙

The use of medicinal herbs has been an intrinsic part of postpartum care in cultures throughout the world. As herbalist David Winston mentioned above, herb teas are given for a variety of reasons, including warding off infection, preventing colic, and nourishing the mother and child. Herbs have also been used both internally and topically to reduce bleeding, ease pain from cramping, increase breast-milk production, heal and soothe the perineal area, and relax the mother.

You can find references to traditional herb use after birth in historical and sociological texts, though the ethnobotany is not often specific. According to Carroll Dunham, women in Thailand drink a mixture of tamarind, salt, and water to "strengthen the womb," while women of the Seri Indian tribe of Mexico drink "seep willow tea" to "stop bleeding after birth." The Jicarillo women chew the root of wild geranium to assist in expelling uterine blood—a known action of this highly astringent herb. According to Sally Placksin, herb use was common in Colombia and Jamaica, as it was in Southeast Asia. In Burma, a paste of turmeric is rubbed onto the body to prevent blood stasis and encourage good circulation while expelling the afterbirth blood. Physician Roberta Lee, director of Complementary Medical Education for Beth Israel Hospital in New York City, lived in Micronesia for 5 years, practicing as a community doctor. There, she told me, women were given baths of turmeric paste after birth.

In both Ayurvedic medicine and traditional Chinese medicine, still practiced in India and China, respectively, and increasingly in other parts of the world, herbs are a routine aspect of postpartum care and have been for thousands of years. The herbs have purposes similar to those of other postnatal treatments, and generally work in conjunction with these.

In more than 15 years of clinical practice as a midwife and herbalist specializing in women's health, I have seen herbs contribute to the health of hundreds of women and children. Interspersed throughout this book you'll find specific herbal recommendations for nourishing and healing yourself during the year after birth.

⋇⋯ BATHING ⋯⋇

Bathing is paid particular attention in the postpartum care of many cultures—with taboos and precautions, as well as recommendations for specific herbal healing baths. In several cultures from Jamaica to Colombia to China, women are prohibited to wash their hair for up to 40 days after birth. However, baths are common, sometimes in the river or creek in very warm climates, or, more often, in hot water with herbs added to heal the woman's "birth wound" (Dunham 1992, Goldsmith 1984) and to "release the flow" of breast milk.

The Yamana women of Argentina are said to walk to the sea to wash thoroughly immediately after the birth, and even in a number of very cold climates women have broken the ice in a creek or pond, or have waded into icy cold water to invigorate the circulation just after the birth. This coincides with the belief maintained by many cultures that it is best for the mother to walk around immediately after the birth to prevent clots from forming and to assist in the flow of blood. It is interesting to note that even in our modern hospitals, women who have just had cesareans are helped out of bed within a couple of hours of the surgery to prevent leg cramps. Women who have birthed vaginally, however, are not usually encouraged to get up right away and walk around.

In Ayurvedic tradition, it is recommended the mother have a daily oil massage, and she should "take a regular daily bath with sufficient quantity of tepid water" (Dash 1975). In Jamaica, where taboos against bathing after birth are strong, women squat over buckets of steaming water to heal their perineal areas (Dunham).

Among one tribe of central Africa, the women are said to go to the river after birth, along with the baby and a group of friends. The mother sits with her legs wide open in the water while everyone is "singing and uttering loud, joyful cries" (Goldsmith). In some cultures, however, according to Goldsmith—for example, the Tallensi of Burkina Faso—the use of hot baths was taken to the extreme, with mother and child both being subjected to water that was nearly scalding. Shrieks of pain, rather than cries of joy, were heard, but these were believed to signify that the water was hot enough for the treatment to be effective. After the baths, the mother received a massage. This was repeated two or three times daily for several days in a row, the water temperature being decreased slightly after the first few days, and decreasing in temperature and frequency over the next few weeks.

The most unusual postpartum custom is probably that from the Marquesans of Oceania. In this tradition the mother and father are encouraged to go to a stream immediately after the baby's birth and have intercourse. Older women of this tribe are said to be emphatically in favor of this custom, though it is not followed much nowadays. Sex immediately after birth is the last thing most women actually think of, but according to the elders, it improved pelvic circulation and healing.

⁂ NUTRITION ⁂

Most women in the United States pay little attention to the foods they eat after birth, unless they are breast-feeding, in which case they may avoid foods thought to produce colic in the baby. The foods provided immediately after birth in the hospital are especially devoid of nutrition. Furthermore, many women, as soon as they give birth, want to begin to diet to regain their pre-pregnancy body size, with no regard for the fact that adequate nutrition is important not only for continued reproductive health, but also for the adequate production of breast milk and for emotional wellness.

The lack of attention paid to food and nutrition in the postpartum in this country is in stark contrast to the diets of traditional cultures. I was shocked to discover, in conducting a thorough review of the literature in preparation for this book, how few medical journal articles address postnatal nutrition. Furthermore, the relative vitality of the foods we eat is significantly poorer than that of foods grown, gathered wild, or hunted by peoples living closer to nature.

As David Winston mentions earlier, the Cherokee people, like those in so many other cultures, fed the mother nourishing foods to rebuild her blood and impart strength and energy. Hot soup is especially common cross-culturally (Placksin 2000), and chicken soup is thought by many cultures to have particular value in healing the new mother. According to Andy Ellis, TCM herbalist and acupuncturist and father of three children, food therapies are one of the most important given to women after birth. Cold foods were avoided, and warm, simple soups, gruels, and stews were prepared that contained grains such as rice and barley, small amounts of meat, and root vegetables. Herbs may have been added specifically for the mother. Chicken and eggs are both common foods to give women who have just given birth. A recently published article in the *European Journal of Clinical Nutrition* verifies the iron value of one traditional Chinese meal—chicken and ginger-vinegar soup—made specifically for the nourishment of postpartum women. The article indicates that the consumption of chicken was higher among the population in the study (postpartum women) than in the general population.

General guidelines for eating well after the birth of your baby will be found throughout this book. Eating high-quality, warming, and nourishing foods—especially organic and natural foods—is an important way to continue to take care of your body after birth, as well as to begin building breast milk if you intend to nurse.

❧ VISITORS ☙

I was once told that in Greece, after the baby is born, the whole village comes together to visit the new mother, bearing gifts for the baby. In some tribal cultures in Africa, not to visit the new mother and baby may have been considered a sign of ill will toward one or the other of them. However, in other cultures, visiting was restricted to the immediate family, and perhaps some close women friends. Frequently a sign was placed on the house to alert the community that a baby had been born to that household. This signified to the friends and neighbors that the new mother and baby were not to be disturbed. Relative seclusion of the mother, as described above, may have served to protect the mother and baby from unwanted infection, and allowed the mother to rest and recuperate freely. Clearly, customs about visitors after birth are variable, but one thing is clear: The needs of the mother and baby should be central. All visitors must maintain a respectful attitude toward these needs and to the sacredness of the space surrounding a new mother and her child.

❧ MOTHER-BABY ☙

The book title *Mamatoto* means "Mother-Baby," describing what in traditional cultures was a virtually inseparable relationship. Mother and baby spent the early days wrapped together in warmth, baby nursing freely, mother alternately resting and becoming familiar with the needs of her newborn. Even in cultures where mother-rest customs were not practiced and mother resumed work shortly—or immediately—after birth, baby accompanied his mother or was tended to by a close relative. Baby was "brought to work" with his mother, carefully carried in a sling or pack that enabled the mother to move about at her work freely. The stresses faced today by new mothers who must work out of the home or who live far from extended family support rarely existed for women living in tribal societies and small villages.

However, one aspect of traditional mother-baby care that has been visibly revived in our Western culture is that of the baby carrier. Slings, backpacks, and rebozos can be seen all over the United States, as parents grow to recognize the value to parents and baby not only of a close and active relationship, but also of the convenience to parents and safety to baby of being close to Mom's or Dad's body.

This renewed interest in baby-carrying coincides with a revival in breast feeding in this country. The benefits of these practices are innumerable for the mother, and range from having a healthier baby to losing weight more quickly after the birth due to the high-calorie expenditure involved in producing breast milk. Although the emphasis of this book is on the care of the mother, new-mother care naturally incorporates her concerns about caring for baby; thus you will find mother-baby information throughout.

✿ MEN AND POSTPARTUM CARE ✿

Traditionally, in cultures where extended families remained intact and lived in close proximity to one another, most of the postpartum care was given to the new mother by other women in the family or community. According to Goldsmith, in a few cultures, it was the husband who helped out. Usually these societies were those in which the larger clan unit was in the process of breaking down, or where families were widely separated; in general, however, it was the mother's family who helped her both during the birth and after. As we have seen, however, fathers do often have significant roles as keepers of birth customs—for example, tending the fire that is so central to the fire-rest traditions.

We also have to look at the lack of centrality of the father's role in relationship to postpartum care in the context of traditional cultures in which monogamous marriages may not have been customary, and where male-female relationships may have held very different meaning from today's marital relationships. In nuclear families, particularly when they are somewhat socially isolated from the extended family, the husband and wife frequently assume for each other many of the roles previously provided by larger family networks. Furthermore, the evolution of the role of women in society has led women to expect more from relationships with men than might have been expected in the past. At the same time, the evolution of the culturally accepted male role to include softer emotions and domestic involvement has changed the nature of the father's involvement in the childbirth process. In addition, social mores about privacy and women's bodies have been somewhat deconstructed. Men in this country are generally more comfortable with the realities of menses, postpartum bleeding, and discussing perineal soreness than were their fathers and grandfathers, thus opening the door for greater ability to provide postpartum support to the mother.

Historically, men had little involvement in the intimate care of the mother in the postpartum process; however, now he may assume much of the responsibility. The potential for closeness and growth for a couple is great when the partner is intimately involved in postnatal care. The potential for stress when the couple does not have extended support is also very great. We will explore these issues in future chapters.

❧　BRINGING THE BEST TO THE WEST　❧

We have a rich and privileged opportunity to learn from the practices of our sisters around the globe and across the centuries, and to incorporate the healthiest practices from other traditions into our own, learning new ways to nourish and support women as they step into motherhood, and bringing new meaning to the days, weeks, and months after the baby is born.

The next chapter outlines how to set up a supportive postpartum situation for yourself *before* your baby is born.

THREE

Preparing for the Postpartum before Baby Is Born

There are few societies in which a single adult is responsible for the care of her babies and other children. Generally, support networks of friends, relatives, hired help, and, in some countries, even government-sponsored assistance are available to the mother to help smooth her transition and also to prevent the burden of care from falling solely on the new mother and father. This allows parents more time and peace of mind for savoring the early days with their baby and enjoying the elation that comes with a healthy birth and baby, an experience that is not repeated many times in the span of a lifetime, and which is not easily recaptured.

Furthermore, in other societies it is rare that a woman giving birth has never herself been involved in helping with another's birth or the care of young children. Extended family means that the mother herself probably has had ample opportunity to look after a younger sibling, niece, nephew, or cousin. Young women, therefore, are frequently realistic about the amount of time and energy a newborn or young child demands.

In the United States, however, most women find themselves isolated at home with their newborn only days after they've given birth, with little prior "on-the-job" experience. Some are single mothers; others are women whose husbands have returned to work. Some of these women are recovering from a cesarean section, which is major abdominal surgery. As 25 percent of all births in the United States are by cesarean, this is a common situation. Many couples live a great distance from extended family when they begin their own family, and because the generation of women who are our own mothers are likely to have jobs or busy lives, it may be difficult for them to get time off to help us for any length of time. Similarly, friends may be busy with their own jobs and families, making help hard to come by if it is not carefully planned for in advance. In many households, a new father may take several days off after the birth, only to return to work full time on a sleep deficit and return home at the end of the day with the full share of household responsibilities. All of this can put tremendous strain on new parents.

Some new parents think they can handle the postpartum by themselves—after all, how much work can a 7-pound person be? While some couples may, in fact, find the transition to parenthood very easy, and may breeze through the learning curve and increased responsibilities of caring for a new-born, such couples are rare. Most need help.

It would be ideal if our customs automatically included new-mother care as part of having a baby. Regrettably, this is not the case; thus, if we are to have postpartum support, we often must arrange it for ourselves. Fortunately, nature provides us with a perfect opportunity to prepare for motherhood—9 months of pregnancy in which to dream, care for ourselves, and plan. The best way to prevent postpartum burnout, optimizing your ability to enjoy your baby and integrate your transition into motherhood, is to take advantage of this time and plan ahead for your postpartum needs before the baby's birthday arrives.

LATE-PREGNANCY HEALTH IS THE FOUNDATION FOR A HEALTHY BIRTH RECOVERY

Excellent nutrition and adequate rest in late pregnancy improve the likelihood of a smooth birth and easy postpartum. Like any other times in our lives when we are tired or poorly nourished, we are more vulnerable to stress, irritability, depression, further fatigue, and illness. When we're exhausted, small challenges can seem like insurmountable obstacles, and little issues can quickly be blown out of proportion, leading to an emotional meltdown.

Too many women run themselves ragged before the birth, trying to get everything in order for the baby. Considering the need to urinate four times a night and other physical discomforts that interfere with sleep, it is easy to see how women enter birth with a deficit of rest. Add a possibly long—and definitely emotionally demanding—experience of birth to the mix and we have the recipe for women to enter postpartum exhausted.

It cannot be overemphasized: Late pregnancy is the time to begin to plan for your postpartum by resting adequately, eating well, and getting light exercise. Rest enhances recovery and decreases stress. Decreased stress means better family relationships, a supported mother-baby bond, less likelihood of postpartum depression, and reduced incidence of child abuse. Sleep is a hard thing to catch up on with a newborn to care for, so set clear boundaries during late pregnancy and develop a plan to ensure you continue to get your own health needs met after the baby comes. A healthy baby requires a healthy mom, and you, too, deserve good health.

HEALTHY BIRTH, HEALTHY POSTPARTUM

The experience of birth lays the foundation for your postpartum experience. During pregnancy, much of the care you receive—from prenatal examinations to nutritional advice—is geared toward growing a healthy baby, with little regard for the emotional quality of the mother's experience. Hospital-based prenatal classes, supposedly designed to prepare you for a healthy birth, too often prepare you for the plethora of interventions that are part of most births in today's hospitals, with their 25 percent cesarean rates, 95 percent epidural rates, and 99 percent episiotomy rates, not to mention the host of other procedures performed ranging from intrauterine irrigation to vacuum extraction designed to protect the baby from the hazards of birth.

In many ways pregnancy and birth become quantitative experiences— how many grams of protein do you eat daily, how much weight have you gained, what is your uterine measurement, what is your hemoglobin count, what is the baby's heart rate, how many contractions are you having per hour and how long are they lasting, ad infinitum. Little emphasis is placed on the importance of natural birth for the health of both baby and Mom from an emotional, qualitative standpoint, nor are women made aware of how great an impact the emotional and psychological quality of the experience can have on the physical outcome. Women ought to be advised that labor interventions can lead to a host of postnatal discomforts and problems. Yet they are not told that cesarean delivery significantly lengthens recovery time and may also interfere with breast feeding, nor are they informed that it predisposes women to greater risk of infection and mortality. It is not uncommon to hear women tell about a cesarean incision that became infected, requiring drainage and special attention for 2 weeks after the birth. Epidurals similarly increase the incidence of postnatal recovery problems, with a large proportion of women who have epidurals suffering from mild to debilitating backache or headache for up to a year after birth (Kitzinger 1994).

All this adds up to the fact that preparation for a healthy and smooth postpartum recovery should include preparation for a healthy birth. Although not all birth complications and thus not all interventions can be avoided, most can be prevented by a holistic approach to childbirth preparation, including attention to physical, emotional, and psychological aspects of birth and a keen awareness of which interventions are necessary and which are clearly not required. It is also important to have a birth support team that will lovingly but firmly act as both guide and advocate for you to help you achieve your goal of a natural birth. Your mate may be an excellent birthing partner, but he has his own share of vulnerability as you go through birth. Therefore, an experienced labor support person to help you navigate the uncharted territory of your birth experience can have a positive impact on the birth journey. Studies demonstrate that having a supportive female at the birth, whether or not she is trained in support techniques, can improve birth outcome and reduce the frequency of birth interventions.

A labor doula may be just such a person. Many labor doulas have training and experience in techniques to help women get through labor naturally. A labor doula will either meet you at home in early labor and go to the hospital with you when your contractions become more active or will meet you at the hospital and stay with you until you are settled in with your baby and nursing. Doulas do not have any formal training in the technical aspects of midwifery or obstetrics—their experience comes from their own births and hands-on work with friends; yet they can still develop a successful practice. When choosing a labor doula, ask about training, experience levels, and fees. Request references, of course, but also go by your sense of comfort with this woman. Are you relaxed and open with her or do you feel tense, judged, pressured, or otherwise uncomfortable in her presence? Let your gut reactions help you determine whether she is the right labor support for you.

PRACTICING BABY CARE

The idea of practicing baby care might seem silly, but if you've never spent time caring for a baby, a little practice before your own magical bundle is born is not a bad idea. Until as recently as a century ago, most women, by the time they became mothers, had extensive experience caring for babies. They'd seen babies breast-fed and knew that babies could thrive on breast milk. Daily baby-care responsibilities, such as changing diapers and bathing a baby, were entirely familiar to them. Feminism has done amazing things for women, enabling us to move beyond the limited roles that prevented us from doing anything but being mothers; unfortunately, though, with our newfound freedoms, we also lost something. Today many women enter motherhood unprepared to care for a baby. While there has been a renewed interest in breast feeding in recent years, most of us did not see our mothers breast-feed during our formative years, and many women have never seen a baby breast-feeding. I've taught many of my clients to put a diaper on their newborn, how to clip a newborn's long fingernails so she doesn't' scratch her tender skin, and how to hold a baby at the breast.

For those of you who have no experience with a newborn or young baby, there is an excellent solution—spend time helping a friend, neighbor, or relative with a baby. You can even tell her you are trying to gain on-the-job experience. Give the baby a bath, change diapers, practice carrying the baby in a baby sling. Any busy mother would likely love to have the help. You'll probably find that your comfort level with motherhood increases as you look forward to caring for your own newborn.

CONTINUUM CARE

Continuum care, or continuity of care, implies that a single care provider follows the cycles of an individual patient from the beginning to the end of the circumstance requiring care. In midwifery, continuity of care means working with a client throughout the pregnancy, through the birth, and through the postpartum period. This allows a deeper relationship to develop between you and your care provider than would occur if you have multiple care providers at various stages of the childbearing cycle.

When you find a care provider with whom you feel comfortable, continuity of care increases the likelihood that you'll feel open expressing anxieties, concerns, and doubts, and it also increases the likelihood that your midwife will recognize when you're having difficulty and will be able to make suggestions based on her understanding of your lifestyle and preferences. Continuity of care with a single practitioner or small group of practitioners is the ideal childbirth care situation. It is therefore important that you gain a clear understanding of whether continuity of care is provided and that you work with practitioners with whom you feel at ease. For example, can you call your obstetrician, nurse midwife, or midwife several days postpartum to ask a question about breast feeding or perineal care? Will you receive a return call or will you have to set up an office appointment for minor concerns? Can your care provider help with breast-feeding and newborn-care concerns? Or will you also have to enlist the help of a lactation consultant and pediatrician for basic questions? Diversifying your care providers so widely might mean your personal needs won't get met, and that you'll have to do a lot of running around if questions or small but common problems do arise.

❧ THE NEEDS OF NEW MOTHERS ❧

What new mothers really need is a few weeks of personal sanctuary time; spa treatment complete with massage, specially prepared healthy meals, time to rest and relax, soothing baths, time out from daily chores and responsibilities, hours to take in the landscape (in this case, baby), time to journal, time to dream, hours of afternoon naps. They also need an extra pair of hands—someone to run the bath, hand them a towel when they get out, someone to bring water or hot tea, someone to answer the phone, take messages, and screen visitors. We need someone to focus on our needs, physically and emotionally, so we can focus on the needs of our newborns. New mothers need someone who can serve as a combination mother, personal confidante, sister, best friend, personal assistant, wise adviser, cook, massage therapist, and housekeeper. It is unlikely that one person can fulfill all of these roles; therefore, it's best to have a support team made up of people who can each meet some of these needs. Unfortunately, many women have difficulty asking for help, feeling they should be able to do it on their own.

New mothers need time and permission to explore and appreciate the range of emotions they are experiencing—new thoughts, new sensations, old memories (both happy and sad), as well as anxieties and fears. A new mother's emotions are extremely labile—joy can shift to tears, elation to depression. For many women, mother love creates a sense of ecstasy, but as Sheila Kitzinger points out, "There is no way from a mountaintop except down." It is natural, as the endorphins and adrenalin—chemical mediators that course through our systems with the stress and excitement of labor, give us the stamina to birth, and naturally reduce our pain sensation—begin to wear off, that we feel a sense of anticlimax, a bit like let-down after all the preparation for the winter holiday season.

Along with these feelings comes the need for a supportive and understanding companion who will listen and validate your feelings. Ideally, your partner will provide some of this support, but he might not fully comprehend the range of your emotions, nor appreciate how you could feel anything but overjoyed by your baby. Therefore, having another woman who has borne children, and who is emotionally sensitive, and with whom you feel you can be open, is sometimes necessary. Another mother can best understand that human emotions are complex, and that we can at once feel unprecedented love and deep anguish, incredible gratefulness and disappointment, deep appreciation and resentment. A good listener and experienced wise-woman can help us put into perspective our emotions, giving us the encouragement to embrace our wholeness as women who are mothers.

When planning for the type of care you want after birth, consider that as a new mom you'll need the following:

- ✑ A good listener whom you can talk to about anything, as many times as you need to, and confidentially
- ✑ Time and space for solitude and reflection
- ✑ Someone who is willing to guard your privacy
- ✑ To feel protected, honored, and nurtured
- ✑ Reassurance that you are doing a good job
- ✑ Noncritical support and advice
- ✑ Praise and encouragement
- ✑ Time-out now and then for a bath, a shower, or a quiet moment
- ✑ Good, healthy food
- ✑ Plenty of rest
- ✑ Respect for your emotions

LEARNING TO ASK FOR HELP AND ACCEPTING IT

Supermom is a fairy-tale character. Real women have the right to ask for help and deserve to receive it. Sally Placksin, in her book *Mothering the New Mother*, quotes one mother as astutely saying, "We gave it away when we said 'I don't need anything, don't come over, I can do it myself.'" Many career women and women having babies later in life have, in fact, been "doing it all," and think this ability can automatically be applied to motherhood. Too often these moms are in for a rude awakening. Indeed, feminist thought should teach young girls that we have the right to have help rather than feeling that we have to do it all on our own.

Realistically, women should think ahead to the first 6 weeks after birth as time to recuperate and heal, then allow another 6 weeks to slowly resume former responsibilities. But many women find it difficult to admit they need help, as if needing help is somehow admitting defeat or saying they're having a problem coping with their responsibilities. It should be just the opposite: Asking for help should be seen as a sign of a healthy and realistic perspective on motherhood. Prenatally, women must develop a sense of rightness about asking for and receiving help after birth. If they wait until after birth to try to access the support they need, it may be too late to coordinate it.

There are numerous reasons that women don't ask for help: Many don't realize they'll need it; most don't want to impose on others; some don't want to give up their privacy by having "help" in the house; some admit that asking for help brings up feelings of failure; others are just too embarrassed or shy to speak up about their needs. Women need to look deep within themselves and sort out conflicting feelings that may prevent them from accessing help, and then seek out the type of help that is most appropriate.

How can you get comfortable asking for and taking help? First, realize it is normal, natural, and healthy to need it. Being realistic is an important sign of being a mature adult. Next, understand that you are not only empowering yourself by asking for help, but are also setting a positive example for other women in your life, who in their own turn might need help. Then realize that taking help and eventually returning help establishes an important basis for community and deep and lasting friendship. Sally Placksin reminds us that it is okay to "owe" people, as it opens us up to our own vulnerability and the softness we experience as new mothers. Receiving help from our friends makes them feel useful, important, and special. It also sets up a situation that allows them to ask us for help in return, and thus reinforces a mutual network of support.

When one of my dear friends went into labor with her second child, my husband drove me to her house (because I was 8 months pregnant myself) to help her with the birth of her daughter—a planned home birth. I returned to her house several days in a row to bring food, check on her, and look in on her older daughter, then 5 years old. Eight weeks later, when I gave birth to my second child—my first daughter—this woman was the first visitor. Lisa brought us dinner, helped clean up after our home birth, and eagerly listened as I poured out the magnificent details of our birth. We nursed our babies together and marveled at the magic of having been pregnant together and of now sharing in the precious beginnings of our children's lives.

Several weeks after my third baby was born, when my husband had to return to work, this same dear friend, now living in another state, brought her girls, by then 9 and 4 years old, by train to my home to stay with us for 5 days, cooking, cleaning, and having woman-to-woman time. This was a precious gift, and one I am grateful I received. While time and distance have lessened the daily intensity of our friendship, there is nothing I wouldn't do to help her or any member of her family.

✣ CREATING A SUPPORT CIRCLE ✣

Everybody loves a newborn, but you'd be surprised how few people ask if they can do anything to help once the baby is born. Friends and family may be busy, and those who don't have children probably have no clue you actually need help. Most women find they actively need to seek out a group of support people for after the birth. Yet it may be awkward to ask people to come to your home to watch your older kids, run a load of laundry, bring a meal, or watch the baby while you grab a nap. More often than not, new moms end up entertaining visitors who come to see the baby, and forgo their own care.

Perhaps the least uncomfortable way to establish a support network is to ask one close friend to be your postpartum support coordinator. It is usually not awkward to call people to ask for help for someone else—in fact, it will probably make your friend feel elevated to a pretty important status in your life. And people do like to be helpful—they just need to be asked and given specific tasks. It would be your job, along with your postpartum coordinator, to brainstorm the areas in which you think you'll need help, then let the coordinator come up with specific assignments for people. The coordinator should provide a master list and phone numbers to each person who is willing to help, so if something comes up and anyone needs to switch her dinner night or afternoon with your toddler, she can call the coordinator or another person on the list.

When our kids were small, we had a children's music tape with a song that had the following chorus: "Some kind of help is the kind of help that helping's all about and some kind of help is the kind of help we all can live without." I think this really sums up the nature of postpartum support, and lays out the importance of being thoughtful about whom we choose to invite into our intimate space at a time when we are establishing our role as a mother and our relationship with our baby. While it is true that new mothers really do benefit from an extra pair of hands around the house—and even a good shoulder on which to laugh and cry—we are also extremely sensitive to discord and vulnerable to criticism during this emotionally open time.

It is easy to create a visual image of a circle of support—your favorite and beloved friends and family members surrounding you and gazing fondly at you and baby, sharing in your joy, and lending a helping hand. But whom do you really want in this circle of support? Bing and Colman suggest the idea of concentric circles of support, rather than one large circle or an amorphic support network. Concentric circles allow a small group of people to be your closest helpers while those who are less intimate but whose help you still welcome are in wider circles that are not as close to you.

The following discussion reviews some of the care options that are available to you after birth. As you review each option, keep in mind the questions listed above to ask yourself to help determine which care options will best serve you. Remember, you can enlist help from several sources, each different choice meeting different needs.

HUSBAND/PARTNER

Your husband or partner is probably your first choice for intimate postpartum care. This is the person with whom you share your daily life, so it's no big deal for you to bare your emotions—or your bottom, as you ask for help in the bathtub or shower. You'll generally feel the safest expressing your vulnerability and will get the most pleasure from enjoying the baby together. The fact that you live together, of course, lends for obvious convenience when it comes to round-the-clock help! It is therefore ideal for your partner to plan to be home full time for at least the first 3 days after birth, preferably 5, if this is your first baby, and for the first week if you have older children who need attention.

Remember that your partner may also be tired after the birth, particularly if the labor was long. However, even if the labor wasn't particularly arduous, he has likely shouldered a considerable amount of anxiety and stress in anticipation of the birth. In letting go of this, he may also need some time to regroup his feelings and energy. New dads are also going through their own feelings about being fathers, which can carry a variety of emotional baggage, depending on his own experience of being fathered. Furthermore, he may see you in new and profoundly different ways now, and his sense of responsibility to his growing family can be overwhelming. All in all, he might need some support, too, and may not be as quickly responsive to your needs as you'd like. He also can't entirely understand the feelings you're going through, either emotionally or physically, as you recover from birth, your hormones skyrocket and plummet, and you integrate your experience of birth and new motherhood.

Ideally, then, you will have time home together during the first few days, with enough help so that Dad doesn't have to prepare all of the meals, care 100 percent for older kids, try to meet your needs, help with the baby, and have no time left to just enjoy and integrate these new relationships. How to avoid paternal overload? It's great to have meals from the freezer that were prepared during pregnancy for this occasion, whether by you or by friends, or to have close friends or family bring in food. This doesn't mean you eat with friends and family—it means they drop off the food, with just a quick hello and good-bye. There will be time for visiting in a few days, and time for sharing meals in a couple of months. Now is the time to create a special aura of protection around your immediate family, with as few interruptions as possible. This creates the ultimate family-bonding experience.

After the first few days or a week, the new dad will probably have to return to work. It is best if this can be done gradually, with him having the flexibility to take off some afternoons or go into work late during the next couple of weeks. If this isn't possible, it's important that he arrange for substitute help whom his wife feels comfortable with. While she may feel ready to be up and around, resuming former responsibilities after a couple of weeks, this is really a recipe for burnout, increased bleeding, and sometimes mastitis for a lot of women. New mothers must be reminded to take it easy, and also need the help that enables them to do so. For the dad to arrange to be off work at 3 o'clock to pick kids up from school, give them a snack, and pay them some attention eases a burden of anxiety and work off his wife, and prevents her from having to run around with the baby. If Dad can't do this himself, he should arrange for a relative or friend to fill in.

Men, remember that your baby and wife will go through peaks and valleys of adjustment during the first several months after birth, so be sensitive to this even if you don't quite understand it. For example, most babies sleep a lot during the first couple of weeks after birth—ironically, the time when women receive the most postpartum help. After 2 weeks, a baby will often start to act more needy, or even fussy. Colic, for example, often doesn't even start for a couple of weeks after birth. So just when you thought it was safe to go back to work, your wife has sleepless nights, finds it harder to calm the baby, and has new things to be anxious about. You, too, may be more exhausted if your sleep has been disturbed by the baby (which it should be if the baby has been up at night!), so fuses may run short and tensions high. Remind yourself to breathe deeply and be patient. You'll both need to work together to find creative ways of coping with stresses, and ask for help from others.

Many couples also find that this is a good time to hire short-term help for things like housecleaning and childcare. (This will be discussed later.)

Husbands need to be extra sensitive and supportive of their wives during this time. It is hard for a dad to know the intensity of emotions that a new mother feels, as not only her hormones but also her body and whole identity go through a shift. Men will get brownie points in the Husband's Hall of Fame if they are kind, gentle, helpful, and supportive during this time—especially without being asked!

OLDER CHILDREN

The surest way to foster a healthy and easy transition for older children, particularly those children aged 2 years to 10 years old, as you welcome a new baby into the family is to prepare them in advance. Watch videos about birth and babies, spend time around friends or family with babies, hunt out opportunities at the playground or in your community to be around babies. Talk about becoming an older brother or sister and what that means. Allow opportunities to arise during which your child can express fears or concerns about the baby or about his place in the family now that there is another sibling coming. Reassure your child that you have more than enough love for all of your children and that he is just as special as ever. Prepare your child for the fact that after the baby is born you will need to rest more for a while, and that new babies demand a lot of holding, feeding, and attention, but giving this doesn't mean you love the older child less. Let him choose new storybooks, crayons or colored pencils and a sketchbook, or quiet games that can be self-engaging or that you would be able to participate in with the baby in your arms. Put these away for "special times" after the birth.

Involve your child in the pregnancy. Allow her to come to prenatal visits and feel the baby's position and listen to the heartbeat. Let her come up with a nickname for the baby, and engage older kids in preparing for the baby's arrival. By the time the new baby is born, her presence will already be an established reality in your older child's life. Older children love to help and feel important. And you'd be surprised how helpful a child of 5 or older can be in small ways, such as handing you a diaper or baby outfit and bringing you a glass of water. If the sibling is old enough, he or she can often safely watch the baby while you grab a shower or fix lunch. He or she will probably beam at being considered responsible enough to help, and this adds positive adjustment to becoming a brother or sister.

If this is not your first baby, you'll probably need some help with the older children, and they'll enjoy getting out of the house a bit too. Arrange for occasional childcare with their favorite people, allowing enough time for the older siblings to enjoy and bond with the baby but enough time out so that you can relax and begin to get to know this newborn. You don't want to create a situation in which older siblings feel unwanted or shuttled off, so be thoughtful to make a balance between home time and away time. Remember, they also may be feeling emotionally vulnerable, have fears or anxieties about your well-being or their place in the family, and also be particularly vulnerable to catching a cold due to increased stress. So love them up, and let them know you care and that they are important. Many families like to have a special gift on hand for older children, to let them know they are special, too. If you're creative in picking a gift, you'll come up with just the thing to occupy them for a couple of hours while you take a nap or are nursing the baby.

RELATIVES

Our own moms are generally the most likely candidates for help during the postpartum. Sharing this time with your mom can be meaningful to both of you, and can help your mother establish a special bond with her grandchild. But for many of us, our relationship with our mother is not all roses. This can lead to challenges for you if you choose to have your mother as your primary postpartum support person. Our own mothers, well intended as they are, have their own agendas, motives, and ideas of how things should be. Your mom may have very different ideas about mothering, and if she is critical or controlling, this will lead to your feeling belittled, stressed, or incompetent. You may also end up angry and resentful. If your mom does not have a good relationship with your husband, this can also be stressful for you, for him, and for your relationship as new parents.

Let's hope your mother is sensitive to the needs of a new mom, and is confident and calm enough in herself to realize that you need support as you figure out how to be a mom. Let's hope, too, she will offer only well-timed, constructive, and gentle advice. But it may be hard for your mom to accept that you are also a mother now, not just her daughter, and that you need space and support to figure out your own way of doing things, as does your husband. Your mom may feel shut out, jealous, or unneeded. As she sees you moving into your own place as a woman and mother, it is possible that she'll exhibit less than supportive behaviors. Women need to be mothered, but they also need to embrace their own empowerment and role as mother during this time.

Sometimes our own mothers cannot provide us with the help we need based on their own experiences. They themselves may have barely been conscious for the birth, only to have the baby brought to them hours or days after you were born. She may have had an extended hospital stay or a visiting nurse who helped at home after the birth. She may have had her own mother to care for her, or she may have had very little care at all. Her own experiences of motherhood, as well as her own experiences as a woman and wife, will have shaped her expectations of how you should care for your baby.

Furthermore, she may have had no exposure to the style of parenting many couples now adopt, which is more baby centered. Most of our mothers were taught to let the baby cry himself to sleep and not to spoil him with too much holding. Most of our mothers did not breast-feed. Therefore, they may have little information to offer us if breast feeding isn't going easily, and if we are exhausted from being up at night with a crying baby, we may be scolded for not just putting the baby in the crib and letting him cry until he falls sleep. We may feel confused as we try to figure out what is right, caught among our emotions and instincts and our mother's advice.

If you have a great relationship with your mom, and she is actively supportive of your choices, this is truly something to be thankful for. Her help will be a welcomed blessing. An extended visit may be just the right thing, especially if she is close with your older children and can help you with them. Make sure she knows you don't plan to run around or entertain while she visits—that you really want her help with the household and your needs, so you can take care of the baby and yourself. Her job is not to take care of the baby so you have a break. If you allow this to happen, you'll miss out on the critical experience of learning to care for your baby from the beginning, and you may feel overwhelmed when Grandma leaves. Furthermore, to establish a successful breast-feeding relationship, the baby needs to be primarily in your arms. You will also want to be clear with your mom that even though you are glad she is there to help, you also need intimate time with your husband and new baby alone. She will have to find ways to occupy herself occasionally so you can have the privacy of being a new family.

Should your relationship with your mom be less than great, and she lives at a distance, defer the visit until after the first week or so, when your hormones begin to stabilize a bit and you're becoming more familiar with the baby. Encourage her to come and help, but keep the visit to a few days. She can always come again when you're more grounded and less susceptible to stressful influences.

FRIENDS

We all have friends with whom we are intimate, and with whom we share a great degree of our personal lives. Similarly, we are likely to have friends whom we can ask directly for help, or who might offer it without our even asking. However, even people with whom we are not close might want to come see the baby. It is perfectly reasonable to be strict about this and delay visits with these friends until after the first few weeks. And if we have friends who share different values about parenting and baby care, and who might be critical or judgmental, it's best to delay their visits as well.

During the months of pregnancy and postpartum, you may receive more from friends than you are able to immediately return. This is okay—nothing to feel guilty about. Good friends operate on a basis of give and take, knowing it all comes out even in the end. In fact, part of the definition of a close friendship is an even exchange. A friend might be cooking for you now, but in a year she could have a baby—or just the flu—and you'll be cooking for her. This is what friends are for. Gratefully accept the help and let your friend know in simple ways how much it means to you.

Sometimes motherhood changes friendships. When I began having kids before most of my friends, their lack of experience in this arena made it difficult for them to offer useful emotional support—they just didn't understand what I was going through. Their childless lifestyles didn't work for me, and my constant preoccupation and distraction because of my children's needs didn't always work for them. Some of those friendships now consist of a call once a year or so; others were revitalized and are stronger than ever because those old friends now have children.

Some friendships simply shift over time as you realize you have different parenting styles. You may find them unsupportive or judgmental as you continue to breast-feed your child into toddlerhood, or they may judge you for choosing either to stay home full time or to go back to work. Mothers with jobs outside the home naturally seek other mothers in a similar situation, just as full-time moms gravitate toward each other as they seek companionship for themselves and their children during the day. You may form new social groups that better meet your needs and have your same interests. This is natural. There is an old expression that says "Make new friends but keep the old; one is silver and the other gold."

MOTHER-TO-MOTHER CARE

An excellent way to create a network of support is through mother-to-mother care. This works best through childbirth classes where women are at differing stages of their pregnancies. Each couple can agree to support the other couples or mothers in turn as they have their babies, bringing food or offering some household help. Of course, the couples must be relatively comfortable with one another. This provides the still-pregnant women with exposure to the mom and newborn after the birth, and has the potential to set the stage for continued support as the children grow older. These families, if they live in reasonably close proximity to one another, often form the basis for a playgroup, mothers morning-out group, or moms support group. These relationships have the potential to grow or just to be helpful in the immediate period when each couple is in the midst of childbearing.

DOULAS

Some parents, particularly those who are accustomed to "doing it all," just don't feel comfortable asking for help. They prefer to hire someone to meet their postpartum-care needs. Some women live too far from family, or don't have enough family or friends in their community to provide adequate postnatal help. A postpartum doula may be the perfect postpartum professional for you. Labor doulas, discussed earlier, provide help during labor; another type of doula, the postpartum doula, provides in-home care after birth. The word *doula* comes from the Greek word meaning "slave," or "handmaiden." Nowadays *doula* has come to denote a woman who helps other women with emotional support and caring for children and household needs. The current usage of the word arose from the work of anthropologist Dana Raphael, who introduced the term in the 1980s after learning the Greek word.

The place of the doula, along with that of childbirth educator, labor doula, lactation consultant, and other professional groups of women helping women in the childbearing year, is a direct testimony to the fact that women need more care, and care of a type different from what is provided by our customary childbirth services at the hands of obstetricians and nurse midwives. (Most home-birth midwives directly provide continuity services or make arrangements for them through their practices.)

Beginning in the mid-1980s, postpartum mother-care services began cropping up in major cities around the country, providing in-home help with cooking, cleaning, grocery shopping, looking after kids, and giving new moms nonmedical assistance and advice on such matters as breast feeding and newborn care. Some doulas receive training through classes designed for this purpose; most, however, are mothers themselves who recognize the need for such services and love helping moms and babies start their relationship in a relaxed and secure manner. The average cost of doula services is $500 per week for 5 hours per day of care. Many couples prefer to hire a doula for after the father has to return to work, frequently for the second or third postpartum week, though many also enjoy the services of the doula for the first week after birth.

It would be ideal for the sake of continuity of care if labor doulas were also postpartum doulas, but this often is not the case, requiring you to hire separate support people for the jobs. It is also unfortunate that neither type of doula service is covered by insurance.

Again, I want to emphasize that the role of postpartum help is not to take over the mother's job of caring for the baby. Any postpartum help should focus on taking care of just about everything else so all you have to do *is* take care of the baby—and yourself. When you interview for postpartum doula help, make certain this is clearly understood, and, as with a labor doula, be sure you are comfortable with the person who will be in your home during those intimate postpartum days. Also pay attention to such factors as health and hygiene, and get very specific and reliable references if this person will be helping with your other children. At present there are no regulations regarding doula care, nor are there specific qualifications or restrictions. Always be careful when inviting a stranger into your home.

HIRED HELP

Other forms of hired help include a mother's helper, usually a high school or college-aged young woman who can come into your home after school and help with the older children. This is a great way for you to get a couple of hours of quiet time or catch up on a bit or correspondence or work, and for your toddler to get some focused playtime or your school-aged child to get help with homework. Or you might choose to hire a housekeeping service for one day a week or every couple of weeks to help out. Some families hire a nanny or an au pair, particularly if the mother intends to go back to work shortly after the birth. This may be a secure option for those who can afford it, but remember, there is no substitute for the attention of the mother and the father, especially the mother, in those early months after birth.

❧ PLANNING AHEAD WITH FOOD ☙

It is helpful to have a week or two of meals planned for after the birth. Many couples put food by during late pregnancy, freezing soups and casseroles that can be defrosted as needed. Enlist family and friends for help with this; ask them either to bring food in advance or take on the responsibility for supplying meals during the first few days after birth.

One of the cleverest ways of arranging food for the new family after birth is the "casserole shower." The hostess invites each guest to bring a meal to the baby shower that can go into the expectant mother's freezer, or a promissory note for a meal to be brought to the family after the birth. The hostess should let people know you want healthy foods that are easy to digest and not too spicy, particularly if she knows the new mom plans to breast-feed, as spicy foods may cause colic in a newborn. Along with the hostess, you can even come up with a list of favorite recipes, and give a copy to friends as suggestions.

If this is not your first baby, plan to have on hand a good stock of your children's favorite foods so it is easy for you, your husband, or a helper to provide food for your child with minimal effort. Knowing you thought of them in advance will also help older children feel cared for. Invite them to help you plan by taking shopping trips together before baby is born and let them pick out what they like to eat. Monitor them, of course, to choose healthy foods—the last thing you want is kids who are living on sweets and bouncing off the walls while you try to relax with a newborn!

❧ BREAST FEEDING ☙

Breast feeding truly is best feeding for babies. Pregnancy is the time to read up on baby feeding choices and to learn about the benefits of breast feeding. Spend time around other breast-feeding moms to help you get comfortable with the idea if you're at all hesitant. Think about how you will breast-feed if you plan to return to work outside the home after the baby is born, which many more working mothers are doing. There are numerous excellent books on breast feeding for working mothers, as well as support groups such as La Leche League International. Subsequent chapters will focus on the joys and challenges of breast feeding.

ᕘ MATERNITY AND PATERNITY ᕗ LEAVES

With so many families having two incomes, there is a lot of planning to do when it comes to arranging time off after baby is born. In fact, many pregnant mothers with jobs outside the home wisely take some time off before the baby is due in order to relax for the last couple of weeks of pregnancy, but then worry how this will affect their maternity leave. For parents with one stay-at-home parent, especially when this is the mom, the situation is frequently less complicated, but it is still also essential for the father to have bonding time with the baby during the early days of life. Many women will also prefer to have their husband as primary support during those early and intimate days after birth. Therefore, the father will need to arrange for some time off.

How much time to take off, and when, depends on the size and needs of the family. With a first baby, especially if there is a good network of help from family or friends, your partner may need to take only a few full days off, and then perhaps keep his option of time off flexible over the next few weeks, allowing him to come home early or go into work late on occasion.

When you already have children, your needs will be different. You'll you have to prepare not only for your own considerations, but also for those of your other children. They will have specific emotional needs as they make room for a sibling. Their unique vulnerability may mean they need the special support only their dad can provide. And your responsibilities will have increased as well. The luxury of an afternoon nap or a relaxing bath that you enjoyed after your first baby was born may be harder to come by with other children to take care of, support, and reassure. This may make mean that Dad has to be more flexible and take more time off from work.

Frequently, when arranging paternity leave, fathers will take off 1 or 2 weeks just after the birth. Many of my clients have found it more useful to stagger the time off over the first few weeks or months, retaining the flexibility to be available as the mother's and older children's needs dictate.

Women who have careers but have the option to stay home full time after baby is born may have a lot on their mind as they sort through their decision whether to continue to work. Some know for sure they will remain at home after baby is born. But other mothers are uncertain what they will do. Many mothers don't make a final decision until after the baby is born. Indeed, many mothers who plan to go back to work at 6 weeks or 3 months postpartum find that with the new arrival, they do not want to return to their job. These women might take an unpaid maternity leave extension for 6 months, and then make their decision at that time. Other women, thinking they will stay home full time, realize they are happier with some personal outlet, and choose to return to a job in some capacity. It is best to keep your options open until you are clear about how you feel.

Many women have no choice but to return to work after the baby is born. This can be extremely stressful. Women who want to be home with baby may feel guilty and torn for working, and all working mothers face the worries that arise when baby is in the care of strangers, especially when their economic situation creates limited choices. Finding childcare can be difficult and stressful, and is therefore best begun before the birth. It is also essential to consider, in advance, how you will continue breast feeding while working. Fortunately, because of the increased number of breast-feeding women in the workforce, there is greater support for this choice.

CREATING A POSTPARTUM SANCTUARY

During the early days postpartum with our four kids, we always put a sign on our door to remind people that our home was a special sanctuary with a newborn inside. On the note we asked guests to keep their visits brief, to postpone their visit if they were sick or had sick children in tow (people are often less public-health-minded than we would like to think), and to pitch in with our kids while in our home. This helped us to set the tone for visits. We generally did not see anyone during the first few days after birth, other than the most intimate of friends and our parents.

The time after birth, as we have seen in earlier chapters, is considered sacred to many. Appreciating this period as unique and a once-in-a-lifetime opportunity allows us to slow down from the fast pace of everyday life and take in the magic of what we have been part of creating. It also allows for complete rest, healing, and recovery. Excellent nutrition, adequate rest, and attention to your emotional self reduces long-term health problems for you and promotes optimal wellness for your baby, while building the foundation for healthy relationships.

❧ DRAWING FROM A FULL WELL ❧

When you are overtired, burned out, or drained, it's difficult to have the type of energy you need for your baby and other children, much less for your relationship with your partner. Being a mother means you're always aware of the needs of others. I think some mothers sleep with one eye open to watch over their children at night. Running on empty doesn't serve anybody in the long run, but is easy to do when you spend all your time giving to others. If you are a breast-feeding mother, you are giving not just emotionally; you are actually giving of your body to feed your baby. Too often women develop the mind-set that a good mother gives all and takes nothing for herself. Remember, this is a great cultural fallacy. A good mother gives of herself to her children, but she has to have a self to give. A good mother nurtures herself, develops her own interests, even if in small ways, and grows as a person along with her children. Children don't need us to be their martyrs; they need us to be their mothers. A self-actualized mother sets an example to her own daughters that becoming a mother expands identity, not limits it.

I teach mothers to use the metaphor of drawing from a full well when they're feeling stressed out and haven't been taking time for themselves. In order to fully nourish your family, you must have reserves to draw on—you need to be a full well. Every bit of help you receive adds to your reserves. Planning ahead for postpartum care ensures that you will have the help and support necessary to keep your well full.

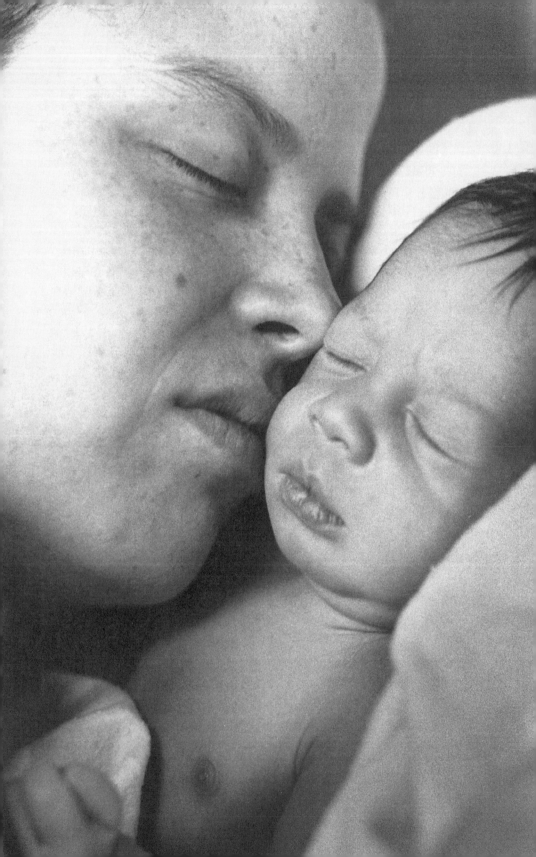

FOUR

The First Days after Birth

*On Crete, right after a baby is born, the mother's breasts and nipples
are washed with chamomile tea before she nurses. When visitors
come to see the new baby, the first question they ask is "has she/he
drunk the chamomile yet?" The tea is considered the perfect thing for
both mother and child after the excitement of labor. Once the baby
has had its first chamomile, it is a huge relief to everyone because it
is a sign that they are healthy and now part of the clan. In the
hospital near the village I live in part of the year, there is a special
room for brewing chamomile for the new mothers and babies.*

Patricia Kyritsi Howell, herbalist

The hours and days immediately after the birth of a healthy baby are nothing short of magical. You watch your baby uncurl from the womb, which had become increasingly cramped quarters for his growing body. Much like watching a time-lapse film of a flower blossoming, the miracle of nature is apparent before your eyes and the beauty of your child at moments will be breathtaking. On the first nights after your baby is born, you might find yourself waking to see if he is really there, or if the birth was just a dream. During those first few days, the endorphins and adrenaline, natural chemicals your body produced to get you through the birth and minimize pain, are still coursing through your body, and you may feel a natural high or euphoria. Every moment is amazing and precious, almost surreal—you just can't believe it's finally happened; your baby has been born.

Along with the euphoria of the first days comes a steep learning curve, particularly if this is your first child. And after a few days, the hormones that create that postbirth euphoria start to decline, often leaving you with a strong sense of anticlimax after the intensity of the birth. Now it's time to chop wood and carry water. Maintaining grace and inner peace as you learn to integrate your baby into your life is possible, and depends in part on your ability to nourish and care for yourself, your patience with yourself as you learn new skills, and getting familiar and comfortable with baby's language and needs. This chapter will guide you through the changes you may experience the first week after your baby is born.

❦　THE BIRTH SETTING　❧

Where you give birth will largely determine your experience in the moments and hours immediately after your baby's birth, as will the nature of the birth itself.

A few of you will choose (and be able) to give birth in the sanctity of your home, and therefore will likely enjoy a quiet, uninterrupted time to relax and enjoy your baby in the comfort of your own bed. Your midwife straightens up from the birth while keeping a gentle but watchful eye on you, and your mother, sister, or friend prepares a meal for you to enjoy. Within an hour or so, you'll probably be in the shower or a soothing herbal bath, and then you'll be tucked into bed to rest with your baby at your side.

For most women, though, the rhythms of a hospital will dictate their immediate postpartum experience. In this case, it will be up to you, your partner, doula, or other labor support person to demand the type of experience you desire. As soon as the baby is born, it is best for both of you to have him placed upon your chest, skin to skin if possible. You must therefore request that the temperature in your birthing room be set to a level comfortable for the baby, as heat loss through the skin can quickly cause the baby's health to become compromised. However, placing the baby next to your skin, with a warm dry towel draped over the baby, in an adequately heated room, is sufficient to ensure the baby's warmth. As long as the baby is pink and breathing well, there is no reason to suspect that the baby needs to be taken out of your arms and placed under a warmer. Note that it is normal for a newborn to have moderately blue hands and feet. As long as the tissue in and around the mouth is not blue, there is no need for worry.

Hospital or birthing center staff may be quite insistent about taking the baby from you to examine him. Unless the baby is clearly in distress, there is no reason to let baby leave your arms. The best place for baby after the birth is near your breast. Any routine examinations can take place in your arms or at your bedside. Unless the baby is ill or struggling, there is absolutely no reason for your baby to be taken to the nursery. Insist that the pediatrician come to your room for the exam, even if the newborn exam needs to be deferred until a pediatrician is available.

During your stay in the hospital, you'll be subject to repeated checks by the nursing staff, and the baby will likely be subjected to a host of interventions unless you protest. Whether to accept vitamin K injections, routine eye prophylaxis with antibiotic ointment, glucose testing, PKU testing, hepatitis B vaccine, placement under a warmer, and formula supplementation of breast milk are just a few examples of the types of choices you will have to make. While law in many states requires eye prophylaxis, it is your choice whether to accept or reject the other options. Therefore, it is important to do research before the baby is born, so you can respond clearly when faced with medical decisions and opinions possibly different from yours.

⅍ BONDING ⅍

Women embrace their babies more or less immediately after birth. Some women fall in love with their babies at first sight, but others take time to feel attached to their newborn. This can be quite normal, but many women feel they are doomed to a poor relationship with their child if they don't bond immediately. This places undue psychological pressures and expectations on women immediately after birth, and interferes with their own intuitive time frame. It is worthwhile to consider where we have come from in the recent history of the mother-baby relationship immediately after birth.

Less than just 20 years ago mothers were still being shaved and prepped for birth with an enema. When the child was "delivered," he was turned upside down by the ankles and spanked, then whisked away from the mother's sight, sometimes not to be seen again by mother for hours. Mother herself may not even have been conscious of the fact that she just gave birth. I can remember births like this when I volunteered at the local teaching hospital as recently as 1984, while trying to get an inside view of hospital births better to inform my practice of midwifery.

I recall an incident from when my children were younger: One spring day I had to pick up a book from a nurse at another hospital, an uptown, upscale facility. As she was a neonatal nurse, my foray took me to the neonatal nursery. My two kids in tow, we peeked into the nursery windows while awaiting the nurse with the textbook I wanted to borrow. My son and my eldest daughter, then aged seven and four, became agitated and my daughter eventually began to cry as we watched the babies in the nursery—all in isolets in a row, and screaming. I think what they found most disturbing was the utter lack of responsiveness from the nurses and pediatrician in the room. My children were accustomed to crying babies receiving comfort and a warm breast. This nursery scene was horrifying to them, and they wanted to leave as quickly as possible. I explained that some people believe that babies can't feel pain or hurt, that they think a baby's crying doesn't mean anything. But my children's empathic response reminded me that human compassion is instinctive: Some humans just seem to manage to block it out with rules and blind customs, especially when it comes to childcare. After all, only recently has pediatric medicine acknowledged that babies are smiling at a few weeks old; it's not that they merely have gas.

We've made some progress in the past decade or so. In the 1970s, pediatricians Marshall Klaus and John Kennell conducted research into the process of mothers "falling in love with their babies," as Sheila Kitzinger puts it in *The Year After Childbirth*. They coined the term *bonding* to discuss this phenomenon, and introduced the term into the medical literature. What mothers have known instinctively and seemingly forever—that the period immediately after birth is a precious and sacred time for the mother-child relationship—now became medical science.

Unfortunately, bonding became the medical expectation. Mothers and babies *should* bond immediately after birth. Ahh, that magic word *should*—a word that can quickly distort a natural and spontaneous experience into a hard-and-fast rule. But the mother-child relationship is also an evolving one, and it doesn't necessarily materialize magically and immediately at birth. Unfortunately for mothers, the imperative for the mother and baby to bond instantaneously became part of the medical protocol in some hospitals and birth centers. Many women who didn't immediately bond with their babies at birth were pathologized—sometimes even observed in the postpartum period for signs of being neglectful or potentially abusive mothers.

Furthermore, many women, aware of the alleged necessity for immediately bonding, began to feel anxious themselves that they were not good enough mothers. A particular incident comes to mind: A client of mine, having been transported to the hospital from a planned home birth, had a truly necessary cesarean section. She saw her baby just after birth, and the father held the baby while Mom was in recovery. She held her baby close soon after the birth, after which baby never left her side. Breast feeding was going very well, and her love for this little one was immense. About a week after the birth, a well-meaning friend gave her a copy of a parenting magazine that promotes natural mothering, which contained an article about bonding. The article expressly stated that C-section moms don't bond as well with their babies as do moms who have birthed naturally. This sent her into a tailspin, with anxiety mounting every time the baby "failed" to make eye contact with her or cried. The mother called me over to observe her connecting with her baby, and the baby acted just like a normal newborn. Mom, however, was a wreck, thinking her birth experience had forever thrust her relationship with her baby into an abyss of disconnection.

It took quite a bit of coaching to help her overcome this doubt, but she did eventually see the narrowness of a view that condemns all mothers who don't birth vaginally to having poor relationships with their children. In fact, it is partially due to the high cesarean rate in our country that bonding at birth hasn't become more institutionalized. One cannot pathologize the 25 percent of women in a society who deliver by cesarean—and immediate bonding after surgical birth can be difficult. So the pressure to bond has fallen by the wayside due to the high rate of obstetric intervention. And so, too, do the high rates of neonatal interventions and "need" for observation of newborns keep the pressures to bond low.

Nonetheless, research demonstrates that women who are given the time to bond with their babies exhibit similar behaviors. They look over their babies from head to toe, coo, talk in high-pitched voices to baby professing their love over and over, and count fingers and toes. And babies, too, come to recognize Mom, by sound and smell especially. Research also shows that the mode of delivery may have an impact on how a woman feels immediately after birth, and thus the ease with which she handles, breast-feeds, and connects with her baby.

What emerges in my mind from all of this research on bonding? Two primary issues seem clear. One is that there is great value in giving mothers and babies time and space to fall in love after birth, whether this takes seconds, minutes, hours, or days. The other is that most of the significant research on postpartum care focuses on the need for the baby to bond with the mother. Indeed, very little research has been done on the needs of the mother postpartum. Yet it seems obvious that the mother's sense of well-being would have an intrinsic influence on her ability and desire to bond with her child. Therefore, it is essential to create a secure, peaceful, supportive, and nurturing environment for the mother immediately after birth, so she has the freedom and opportunity to begin her relationship with her baby right from the start.

❧ PHYSICAL CHANGES IN THE DAYS ❧ AFTER BIRTH

Regardless of where you birth, the changes a woman's body goes through after the birth are similar in all women. Although most women feel elated and want to hold and look at their baby, some women are fatigued and overwhelmed, and want to rest with baby either tucked beside them or in a trusted relative's arms. A meal or snack high in protein and complex carbohydrates, such as eggs and toast, chicken soup, or miso soup with tofu and noodles, along with fresh seasonal fruit, provided about an hour after birth is important for stabilizing the blood sugar and restoring the energy expended during the labor. Protein is also important for healing tissue. Therefore, it is best to eat something even if you are tired and want to sleep.

ACHING MUSCLES

Certain muscle groups that you used during labor—particularly your arms, back, and legs and will be sore. A relaxing herbal bath (see page 89) and a good rest can bring great relief, and you'll welcome a deep massage within a few days after birth.

HEALING TENDER PLACES, TEARS, AND EPISIOTOMIES

Your perineum may be tender. Even if you had no tear or an episiotomy at birth, that tissue had to stretch wide to let your baby through. Sometimes, too, there are very small skin abrasions on the inside of the labia, which midwives refer to as skid marks. These may sting when you urinate during the first few days. Tender care with an herbal bath, herbal compresses, herbal rinses from a peri bottle while you urinate, or an ice pack if you have a lot of swelling, can all be soothing. If you have a small tear and chose not to have stitches, drizzle $1/2$ to 1 teaspoon of vitamin E oil (d-alpha tocopherol) on the tear 2 or 3 times daily to encourage healing.

❧ HERBAL BATHS ❧

There are many herbs that will soothe tender perineal tissue, heal tears and episiotomies, reduce inflammation, decrease hemorrhoids, and prevent infection. They are also calming and nourishing to the mind and spirit. The postpartum bath is a tradition that my clients have enjoyed for 15 years. Purchase and mix the herbs yourself to have on hand after the birth, or purchase premixed herbs (see Resources).

Preparing the bath is as simple as making a giant pot of tea, and the medicinal liquid can also be made into compresses and peri-rinses as directed below. You can take the bath as soon as an hour after birth, then repeat once or twice daily for 3 to 5 days. Let your baby accompany you into the herbal bath, which also promotes healing of the umbilical site.

 Herbal Bath I: Postpartum Delight

This blend of beautiful and fragrant blossoms is uplifting, soothing, healing, and antiseptic.

> 2 ounces comfrey leaves
> 1 ounce calendula flowers
> 1 ounce lavender flowers
> 1 ounce sage leaf
> $^1/_2$ ounce myrrh powder
> $^3/_4$ cup sea salt

Mix together the comfrey, calendula, lavender, sage, and myrrh. Bring 4 quarts of water to a boil. Turn off the heat and place 1 ounce (approximately 1 large handful) of the mixture into the pot. Steep, covered, for 30 minutes. Strain the liquid with a fine-mesh strainer and discard the herb material.

Add 2 quarts of the liquid to the tub, along with the salt. Reserve the remaining liquid for another bath, for compresses, or for a peri bottle.

Herbal Bath II: Deep-Healing Bath

Strongly antiseptic and astringent, this mix is perfect for healing trauma to the perineum, including tears and episiotomies.

> 1 ounce dried comfrey leaf
> 1 ounce yarrow blossoms
> 1 ounce dried sage leaf
> 1 ounce dried rosemary leaf
> 1 large fresh bulb of garlic
> $^1/_2$ cup of sea salt

In a medium bowl, mix together the comfrey, yarrow, sage, and rosemary. Peel all the garlic cloves and place them in a blender with 2 cups of lukewarm water. Blend at high speed until you have a milky liquid and the garlic is completely pulverized. Strain through a fine-mesh strainer.

Bring 6 cups of water to a boil, then turn off the heat. Add 1 ounce of the dried herb blend to the pot and steep for 30 minutes. Strain the liquid and discard the herb material.

Pour 1 cup of the garlic "milk" and 4 cups of the herb tea into the bath, along with the salt. Reserve the remaining liquids for a subsequent bath.

Caution: Do not use the garlic milk in a peri bottle or compress—it would be too irritating. The tea, however, is safe to use in the bath.

FOR AN HERBAL COMPRESS

Simply soak a washcloth in the herbal tea and apply warm or cold to the perineum, as needed, to reduce tenderness and swelling.

FOR A PERI-RINSE

Purchase a peri bottle, a plastic squeeze bottle, from any pharmacy and fill with the strained tea of your choice. Use warm or at room temperature. Squeeze over your perineal area as you urinate. This significantly reduces inflammation and stinging.

 After-Birth Massage Oil

This simple combination, massaged into aching muscles, can bring great relief, whether or not you've just had a baby.

> 3 ounces almond oil
> 1/2 ounce arnica oil
> 1/4 ounce essential oil of rosemary
> 1/4 ounce essential oil of wintergreen

Mix well in a small plastic squeeze bottle and store in a cool, dark place. Apply as needed, shaking well before each use.

AFTERPAINS

Usually within 30 minutes after the birth of the baby, the placenta is delivered, at which time your uterus weighs more than 2 pounds. According to Kitzinger (1994) its weight is reduced by 95 percent over the next 6 weeks. This process, known as involution—squeezing it back into shape and size—occurs through uterine contractions, often referred to as "afterpains" or "after-birth pains." Afterpains generally begin within 12 hours of the birth, and may be quite painful, some women complaining that they hurt more than labor contractions. They frequently occur with increasing intensity with each subsequent baby, as each pregnancy causes the uterus to become slightly more stretched. Although you might not experience afterpains, it is important to be aware that they can occur, lest you be taken by surprise and think something is drastically wrong.

Should you experience severe cramping, don't take aspirin. The purpose of the cramps is to clamp down the uterus, not only restoring it to its original size and shape but also preventing excessive bleeding. This occurs because the uterine blood vessels are interlaced with the uterine muscle fibers. Contraction of the uterine muscle fibers leads to enough constriction of the uterine blood vessels to control bleeding. Aspirin can cause blood thinning and increased bleeding.

Nursing your baby will trigger the cramps because breast feeding also stimulates the release of oxytocin, a hormone naturally occurring in the body that causes uterine contractions (pitocin is synthetic oxytocin), and is an excellent way to speed the process. Therefore, don't be tempted to use a bottle instead of the breast until the cramps pass. They are almost always completely gone by 72 hours after the birth, and often well before that. Doctors sometimes prescribe acetaminophen (that is, Tylenol) or an anti-inflammatory such as ibuprofen. Although these are considered safe while breast-feeding, it is preferable to avoid unnecessary medications. Natural remedies and simple comfort measures can relieve cramps while encouraging uterine tone, thus aiding the body in the involution process. Comfort measures include a warm bath and a hot-water bottle applied to the lower back or lower abdomen. Moxabustion treatments (see pages 48–50) and hot rice packs (see below) can relieve the cramping as well.

HERBS FOR AFTERPAINS

Midwives and herbalists have long prescribed herbs for the relief of afterpains. Try the following if you have bothersome cramps and want a natural therapy. These herbs are not contraindicated for use while breast-feeding (LowDog 2001), and may be considered safe for use.

Chamomile tea (*Matricaria recutita*): Chamomile is a gentle herb for easing aches, cramps, and spasms, and is considered beneficial for supporting breast-milk production. It is calming for the mother and may help prevent or reduce colic in the baby. Put 1 tablespoon of chamomile blossoms in 1 cup of boiling water and steep, covered, 10–15 minutes. Strain and discard the herb material. Drink warm, lightly sweetened if desired.

Catnip tea (*Nepeta cataria*): Catnip shares many of the same principles as chamomile and may be used instead of chamomile or in combination.

Prepare as for chamomile, or to combine, use $^1/_2$ tablespoon of each and prepare as above.

Dose: 1–4 cups daily, as needed

Motherwort *(Leonurus cardiaca):* As the name of this herb implies, it is meant for mothers. *Wort* means "healing herb." The Latin botanical name, *Leonurus cardiaca,* means "lion-hearted," and many herbalists interpret this to indicate that it provides a certain strength and stoutness to the character when there is depression, anxiety, or irritability. It is an excellent tonic for both the uterus and the heart, tonifiying the former and reducing palpitations in the latter. It also takes the edge off spasmodic uterine cramps, making it well placed as a pain-relieving uterine topic for afterpains. It is quite bitter, and is thus better used in tincture form.

Prepare a cup of catnip tea and add 1 teaspoon of motherwort tincture after the tea has been steeped and strained.

Dose: $^1/_2$–1 teaspoon up to 4 times daily

HOT RICE PACKS

Hot rice packs are easy to make, can be used during labor for lower backache, and are effective postpartum for after-birth pains in place of a hot-water bottle.

Method 1: Place enough rice in a long tube sock to fill it two thirds of the way. Firmly tie the top closed with a cotton string and place in the microwave for 2 minutes on medium heat. Apply to crampy areas as needed.

Method 2: Cut a piece of cotton fabric into a rectangle 36 inches long and 4 inches wide. Fold in half so it is 18 inches long and 4 inches wide, then sew together the two long ends with close stitches. Fill two thirds of the way with rice and sew the last side closed firmly. Heat in the microwave and apply as above.

Either sack can be reheated and reused as needed.

Optional: Add $^1/_4$ cup of lavender blossoms to the rice and mix well before placing in sack. When heated, the lavender will emit a soothing and pleasant fragrance.

Note: Severe cramps accompanied by uterine tenderness, fever, or foul-smelling discharge may signal serious uterine infection. Should you experience these symptoms, seek medical care immediately.

SHAKES, SWEATS, AND OTHER BODY QUAKES

During the few days following birth, many women find they sweat profusely, or experience periods of intense shaking, generally from getting chilled as a result of sweating. This is due to hormonal changes and the body's effort to eliminate extra fluids that have accumulated during the course of pregnancy. Similarly, you may have to urinate frequently. Sip warm ginger or cinnamon tea, keep the ambient temperature comfortable, and have a warm blanket and socks on hand if you get chilled. Ask your partner to hold or massage you if you experience shaking. These symptoms will abate quickly on their own, and do not need special attention unless there is accompanying fever or other signs of illness.

GINGER TEA

Place 1 teaspoon of freshly grated gingerroot in 1 cup of boiling water and steep, covered, for 15 minutes. Strain, lightly sweeten with honey, and sip while warm, up to 2 cups daily.

Variation: Simmer 1 teaspoon each of dried red ginseng pieces *(Panax ginseng)* and dried licorice root *(Glycyrrhiza glabra)* in boiling water for 15 minutes. Turn off heat and proceed as above to add the ginger and make ginger tea.

Sip while warm, up to 2 cups daily. This is a more tonifying tea, and is excellent to drink if you experience chills and sweating after the birth.

CINNAMON TEA

Steep $1/2$ teaspoon of cinnamon powder in 1 cup of boiling water for 5 minutes. Sweeten with honey and add milk if desired.

Dose: $1/2$ to 1 cup

A specific traditional Chinese formula for treating severe postpartum sweating is as follows:

30 grams oyster shell

12 grams astragalus

12 grams codonopsis

12 grams ophiopogon

9 grams dang gui

9 grams fu xiao mai ("floating wheat")

9 grams ma huang root

9 grams peony

9 grams rehmannia

6 grams schizandra

9 grams siler

These herbs are used to promote the body's ability to maintain its protective influences *(wei qi),* retain energy, and rebuild fluids. To obtain these herbs, see Resources.

To prepare, take either in prepackaged granules, 6 grams daily, or lightly boil in 6 cups of water for 1 hour. Strain and take $^1/_2$ cup twice daily until the tea is finished. Refrigerate the unused portion and heat each dose as needed. You may leave the daily dose at room temperature and take without heating first.

BLEEDING

If there is excessive bleeding to the point of a hemorrhage immediately after the birth of the baby or the expulsion of the placenta, your doctor or midwife may give you an intramuscular injection of pitocin to stop it. Continuous or heavy bleeding anytime in the first week after birth should be immediately reported to your care provider. It is normal to experience anywhere from 2 to 6 weeks of bleeding, known as lochia, during the early postpartum. This is caused by a shedding of the endometrium, the lining of the uterus, which builds up during pregnancy to provide a bed of rich nourishment for the baby via the placenta.

The intensity and duration of the bleeding depend primarily on uterine tone and your physical activity level. The more toned your uterus is, the lighter and shorter the duration of bleeding is apt to be. Moderate to excessive activity is likely to cause an increase in your bleeding. Immediately after birth, a full, distended bladder will prevent your uterus from contracting effectively, and may contribute to a continued trickle of blood. Unchecked, this can lead to significant blood loss. Be sure to get up and urinate within a couple of hours of the birth to minimize the possibility of excessive postpartum uterine bleeding.

During the first 3 to 5 days after birth, bleeding should be like a moderate to heavy menstrual period. You may also pass clots of varying sizes, even occasionally as large as an egg. This is usually because blood pools up in your uterus while you are reclining and clots, then is passed when you stand up or use the toilet. To minimize the formation of clots, firmly massage your abdomen periodically and each time before you stand if you've been lying down, until you feel your uterus become hard like a small cantaloupe or grapefruit. Your midwife or doctor can show you how to do this a few hours after the birth. By the third day postpartum your uterus will have begun to shrink enough that this is unnecessary. Wearing an abdominal binder also wards off clots and excessive bleeding.

After this time the bleeding will lighten to a watery brown color, and gradually, over the next weeks, will become even lighter and then stop. Significant activity, lifting, and pushing motions can cause the bleeding to resume, and postpartum hemorrhage can still occur up to 30 days after the birth. Therefore, be cautious doing strenuous activity, heavy lifting, or chores such as grocery shopping and vacuuming during the first 4 to 6 weeks. During the first week, don't lift anything heavier than your baby, and keep physical activity and exercise to a minimum.

During the first few weeks postpartum, avoid tampons, as they might increase the risk of infection. Similarly, it is not a good idea to use cloth reusable pads or menstrual sponges. The most hygienic sanitary product to use during the first 10 days postpartum is disposable, unbleached menstrual pads. These decrease the risk of infection. During the first week you'll need maternity-size pads, and you'll probably even need to double them up at night. After that, you can switch to maxi pads and then down to thinner pads.

It is important to keep up iron-rich foods during the first weeks after birth to compensate for blood loss and to prevent iron-deficiency anemia. Foods high in iron include red meat, dark-meat turkey, red beans, lentils, dark green leafy vegetables (such as kale, collards, and broccoli), and dried fruits such as raisins, black mission figs, apricots, and cherries.

Herbal Treatments for Postpartum Bleeding

In the literature of the Eclectic physicians—doctors who practiced from the mid-19th to the early-20th century and used botanical medicines widely in their practices—as well as the traditions of midwives from Europe, there are numerous references to herbal remedies for uterine bleeding (Ellingwood 1919, Felter 1922, Felter and Lloyd 1898, Fyfe 1905). The action of many of these herbs is primarily to bring tone to the uterine tissue. Toned uterine muscle prevents excessive laxity of the uterine blood vessels, and hence prevents excessive bleeding.

Although in emergency situations such remedies should be used only by trained practitioners, you can try them for normal but heavy postpartum uterine bleeding. Here are some herbal formulas that are safe to use to help diminish heavy postpartum uterine bleeding from poor muscle tone.

 Lady's-Mantle Blend

See pages 242–44 to learn about tinctures.

> $1^1/_2$ ounces tincture of cotton root *(Gossypium herbaceum)*
> 1 ounce tincture of lady's mantle *(Alchemilla vulgaris)*
> $^1/_2$ ounce tincture of shepherd's purse *(Capsella bursa-pastoris)*
> $^1/_2$ ounce tincture of cinnamon *(Cinnamomum zeylanicum)*
> $^1/_2$ ounce vegetable glycerin

Combine the tinctures in a 4-ounce bottle, then add the glycerin.
Dose: $^1/_2$–1 teaspoon as needed until the bleeding stops, up to 8 teaspoons

 Yarrow and Shepherd's Purse Tea

> $^1/_2$ ounce dried shepherd's purse herb *(Capsella bursa-pastoris)*
> $^1/_2$ ounce dried yarrow blossoms *(Achillea millefolium)*

Combine the yarrow and shepherd's purse. Steep 4 tablespoons of the blend in 2 cups of boiling water, covered, for 20 minutes. Strain and discard the herb material.
Dose: $^1/_4$ to 1 cup as needed, lightly sweetened, if desired, up to 4 cups

 Cinnamon and Erigeron Formula

Based on the prescriptions of Dr. Ellingwood, this formula will quickly stanch heavy postpartum bleeding. If bleeding persists, seek medical advice. This formula is available from Herb Pharm (see Resources).

> $1^1/_2$ ounces tincture of Canada fleabane *(Erigeron canadensis)*
> $^1/_2$ ounce tincture of cinnamon *(Cinnamomum zeylanicum)*

Blend the tinctures well.
Dose: $^1/_2$ teaspoon as needed, up to 6 doses over 2 hours

Note: Midwives and obstetricians insist that if you soak more than two large menstrual pads in 30 minutes, this constitutes a hemorrhage and requires medical attention. Passing large clots, or continuous bleeding even if only moderate but accompanied by abdominal tenderness, fever, or foul-smelling discharge, could indicate retained fragments of the placenta or amniotic membranes in your uterus, possibly with infection. Should you experience these symptoms, seek immediate medical attention.

TREATING HEMORRHOIDS

Hemorrhoids can be a real pain in the . . . well, you know. Unfortunately, for many women they are a fact of life after birth, particularly if they were already a problem during pregnancy, or if there was a long pushing stage at birth. The good news is that simple home treatments can effectively reduce them and the discomfort they cause. In general, if hemorrhoids are a problem you want to avoid constipation. You should eat a diet high in fiber, including fresh vegetables and whole grains. Also, be sure to drink plenty of water.

The following simple treatments can be used directly on the hemorrhoids to shrink them and reduce inflammation.

 Tea Bag Packs

Steep a caffeinated tea bag (any kind, even Lipton, will do) in about an eighth of a cup of boiling water. Let sit for 2–3 minutes. Squeeze excess water from the tea bag and apply the bag directly to the affected area. *Note:* tea stains, so wear a pad when wearing the tea bag. This treatment can be repeated several times a day.

 Bum-Ease

Fill a 4-ounce, widemouth glass jar with round cosmetic pads. Fill the bottle with witch hazel, available at your local pharmacy. You can also add 5–7 drops of antiseptic and pleasantly scented essential oil of lavender. Apply the soaked pads to the affected area, repeating as needed.

ᏄᎬ THE SHAPE OF YOUR BODY ᏄᎬ

Immediately after giving birth, particularly the first time you stand up, you'll notice that your belly has dramatically decreased in size. In fact, standing up for the first time might even cause you to catch your breath or experience a strange empty sensation in your diaphragm. All the pressure that was there from housing your baby just hours ago are suddenly gone. However, your pregnant belly will not reduce in size completely until several months postpartum, and for the first several weeks your belly might still look like you are 5 months pregnant. This is normal, and moderate exercise, a healthy diet, and the caloric output of breast feeding will all help you to regain your shape.

Similarly, your slightly larger hips and buttocks, which have stored fat reserves for nourishing you and the baby, will be noticeable for several months.

Stretch marks begin to fade and turn silvery over the course of the months postpartum, but even within the first week after birth cease to be as prominent as they were in late pregnancy.

It is common for women to struggle with body-image issues during the postpartum. Unfortunately, the cultural stereotype of "thin is ideal" causes us to feel fat and frumpy during the months after birth. It's very important to be honest with yourself about how such an internalized message might be affecting your opinion of your body, because you might unconsciously eat less than you need in an effort to regain your pre-pregnant size. Skimping on meals, however, can lead to depression, irritability, and difficulties with breast-milk production. Furthermore, your body will make what it needs for the baby, compromising you in the process in the form of pulling nutrients from your bones and muscles. As women, we need to learn to resist unhealthy cultural stereotypes, and replace these with pride and gratitude for our own beautiful shapes, whatever they are. This does not mean that you should not eat properly and get moderate exercise. Or that there is anything wrong with being in good physical shape. However, our own body type should determine this shape, not an image on a magazine cover.

❧ HEALING FROM A CESAREAN ❧

Women experience varying levels of discomfort after a cesarean. Regardless of the level of intensity of post-cesarean discomfort, having just had major abdominal surgery requires that you rest more than from a vaginal birth, and also impedes some of your range of motion and flexibility. Therefore, be extra patient and gentle with yourself as you learn to hold, comfort, and feed your baby in a limited number of positions. A nurse, your midwife, or a lactation consultant can help you to find comfortable positions for nursing and resting.

In addition to soreness at the site of the incision, you may experience pain in your abdomen, back, or shoulders from gas pockets that got trapped inside during the procedure. Many women are never informed that this can happen, and thus are unprepared for the sometimes painful gas pains they encounter. These pass quickly on their own, but knowing what they are can spare you panic.

Most often the incision on your abdomen heals without difficulty, but I've seen a number of cases where women developed abscesses at the incision, which opened and drained. To prevent this, keep the site clean and dry, and allow good air circulation and sunlight (lying in front of a window provides adequate light in most climates, and during most times of the year) to reach your belly for at least 20 minutes each day. When you shower, fill a peri bottle with tea from Herbal Bath I (see page 89) and squeeze this over the incision to promote healing and reduce inflammation, soreness, and the risk of infection. Gently pat yourself dry after the shower. It is preferable to wait to take a bath until a week after the cesarean.

POST-CESAREAN PAIN

Many doctors prescribe pain medication to take during the first couple of days after a cesarean, but most breast-feeding mothers would rather not take any medications after birth. There are a few herbal analgesics that are effective substitutes for painkillers. California poppy *(Eschscholzia californica)* and Jamaican dogwood *(Piscidia erythina)* can be taken alone or combined in small amounts with other herbs to reduce or relieve abdominal or generalized discomfort resulting from surgery. They are nonaddictive and are not specifically contraindicated for use while breast-feeding (McGuffin et al. 1997, LowDog 2001, Blumenthal 1998); however, as with many other herbal medications, few studies have been conducted to absolutely determine safety.

The following combinations make use of these herbs in small quantities, along with larger amounts of herbs that have a long track record of use for promoting relaxation in new mothers. Either formula may be taken regularly for 1 week, after which time you should discontinue it. Do not modify the proportions of the herbs in the formulas or increase the dose beyond what is described below.

 Herbal Analgesic I: Eschscholzia *Combination*

Take for pain with inability to sleep. (See pages 242–44 to learn about tinctures.)

> 1 ounce tincture of California poppy *(Eschscholzia californica)*
> 1 ounce tincture of cramp bark *(Viburnum opulus)*
> 1 ounce tincture of passionflower *(Passiflora incarnata)*
> 1/2 ounce tincture of chamomile *(Matricaria recutita)*
> 1/4 ounce lavender *(Lavendula angustifolia)*
> 1/4 ounce vegetable glycerin

Combine the tinctures and the glycerin.

Dose: $^1/_2$ teaspoon up to 8 times daily. Up to 1 dose every 30 minutes for 2 hours to promote sleep.

 Herbal Analgesic II: **Piscidia** *Combination*
For abdominal pain with intestinal gas or discomfort. (See pages 242–44 to learn about tinctures.)

> 1 ounce tincture of chamomile *(Matricaria recutita)*
> $^1/_2$ ounce tincture of hops *(Humulus lupulus)*
> $^1/_2$ ounce tincture of lemon balm *(Melissa officinalis)*
> $^1/_4$ ounce tincture of Jamaican dogwood *(Piscidea erythina)*
> $^1/_4$ ounce vegetable glycerin

Combine the tinctures, then add the glycerin.
Dose: $^1/_2$ teaspoon up to 6 times daily

❧ YOUR DIGESTIVE SYSTEM ☙

In addition to nesting instincts that cause you endlessly to clean your house in late pregnancy, many women experience a physiological "housecleaning" in the few days or couple of weeks before birth in the form of more frequent or looser bowel movements. This is partly a result of increased hormonal activity, which creates more relaxation of the bowels, and also a result of having less room in there because of increased pressure from the baby on the digestive system. Some women also have increased bowel activity during labor. After birth, it is normal not to have a bowel movement for 24 or even 48 hours. To prevent constipation, eat soft and easy-to-digest foods for the first couple of days, as well as adequate fiber. Be sure to drink ample water, at least 8 glasses per day. Neither over-the-counter laxatives nor stimulating herbal laxatives (senna and buckthorn, for example) are recommended while you are lactating. However, you can use bulk laxatives such as psyllium seeds, as well as soaked or stewed dried fruit and bran, should constipation be a problem. Below you will find two gentle laxative recipes.

Some women become slightly constipated after the birth because they are afraid to have a bowel movement. This is particularly the case for women who have had an episiotomy or a cesarean. Keeping your bowel movements soft, as directed above, and relaxing while you have a bowel movement to help you avoid straining will make things easier, but remember, episiotomies and cesarean repairs are meant to withstand such normal physiologic functions.

For the Treatment of Mild Constipation

These are safe laxatives for use while breastfeeding when used as directed. Discontinue after one week if relief is not found and seek the advice of an experienced professional.

 Gentle Lax

This not only helps relieve constipation, but it is nutritious as well.

> ¹/₂ cup warm unfiltered apple juice
> ¹/₂ cup warm water
> 4 prunes
> 2 dried Black Mission figs
> 1 heaping tablespoon bran flakes
> Dash of cinnamon

Pour the juice and water into a medium mixing bowl. Add the prunes, figs, bran, and cinnamon and let soak for 15 minutes.

Take in the morning before breakfast each day as needed.

 Easy Going

Soak 2 teaspoons of psyllium seeds in ¹/₂ cup of unfiltered apple juice for 10 minutes and consume the whole mixture. Follow with a full glass of water.

 Herbal Lax

Place 2 tablespoons each of dried dandelion root and dried yellow dock root in a 4-cup saucepan. Add 2 cups of cold water and gently bring to a simmer. Let simmer, uncovered, for 20 minutes, then strain.

Drink 1–2 cups daily as needed. This can be done in addition to either of the above treatments for more difficult constipation.

❧ WHEN YOUR MILK COMES IN ☙

Late in pregnancy, your body begins to produce a substance called colostrum, which is present in your breasts during the baby's first few days of life. This thick, yellowish liquid is very high in antibodies, and helps to provide your baby with an excellent beginning for her immune system. In addition, the antibodies help the baby colonize the right kind of digestive flora, which leads to a significantly decreased risk of future bowel problems and allergies compared to that of babies who were not breast-fed. Therefore, it is important to let the baby nurse amply during the first few days and not supplement because you think your milk is not in yet. Supplementation for a baby that you plan to breast-feed should occur only if there is a true threat of malnutrition or dehydration for the baby due to actual insufficient quantities of breast milk, which is very rare.

Between 36 and 72 hours after your baby is born, milk will begin to fill your breasts. The true milk is a much thinner substance than the colostrum and is white, perhaps even appearing to have a bluish-white tinge. It is also sweeter than the colostrum. Just prior to or as your milk comes in, you may notice a number of physical and emotional changes, including increased body temperature and even a low-grade fever, breast tenderness, breast engorgement, and weepiness or irritability. Breast engorgement can be significant, with the breasts dramatically expanding several bra sizes. This fullness, which will recur whenever your breasts get very full over the first couple of months, can cause your breasts to feel tight, hard, and uncomfortable. The most effective way to reduce the engorgement is to breast-feed your baby as much and as often as she is willing. However, the fullness of the breasts often also causes the nipples to be pulled tighter and might make it harder for your baby to latch on. In this case, or if the engorgement is extremely uncomfortable and the baby doesn't drain off enough to relieve the fullness, express milk either by hand or gently with a breast pump. You can also try other methods of getting the milk to flow out freely and relieve the engorgement:

- Take a bath or shower and let comfortably hot water run over your breasts. Gently hand-express milk, and when the milk begins to flow, let it do so freely.

- Apply hot compresses to your breasts. First gently rub a thin layer of arnica oil over your breasts (not your nipples), then apply a hot compress to reduce soreness.

- Have your partner nurse to get the milk flowing or reduce the volume (depending on how much he wants to suckle!).

- Apply bruised cabbage leaves to the whole breast. To bruise, place them on a cutting board and roll over them with a rolling pin.

To prevent recurring severe engorgement, let the milk run freely from one side while the baby nurses the other, rather than trying to stop the flow with firm pressure, and allow the baby to nurse freely. Avoid sleeping in a position that puts pressure on the breasts, and avoid constricting bras or other tight clothing, as these all can contribute to clogged milk ducts.

℘ BREAST-FEEDING CHALLENGES ℘ IN THE FIRST DAYS ℘

A lot of women think that because breast feeding is so natural, it must be really easy. However, this is not true in a lot of cases. Breast feeding, although a natural process, also requires some skills learned by both you and the baby. While some babies take readily to nursing, many, if not most, require some coaxing and a lot of patience.

This may sound simple, but if your precious little baby is screaming his head off because he's hungry and frustrated, and your postpartum hormones happen to be swirling around (and likely they will be), you've got a recipe for a panic attack or at least a good cry on your part. The sound of baby's crying is designed to raise your alarm bells: This is the baby's built-in protective mechanism to his lifeline—you—and it works! Your husband may be confused, overwhelmed, and jarred by the baby's crying as well, and you may have the added pressure of a nurse or relative suggesting you just give the baby a bottle so he can calm down, so he doesn't become dehydrated and sick. And all the while you're supposed to be calm and relaxed so the baby feels comforted and so your milk lets down!

Many potentially successful breast-feeding relationships suffer or fail before they've even had a chance due to misinformation or misunderstanding on the part of the parents—and lack of support for getting it right. You can succeed at breast feeding if you remember these thoughts:

- Natural doesn't mean easy.
- You can breast-feed.
- Patience and perseverance will be rewarded with a successfully nursing baby.
- Healthy babies born close to full term rarely become dehydrated or compromised if it takes 2 or 3 days to establish a successful breast-feeding relationship.
- Centering and calming yourself in spite of your baby's mood is essential, even if you have to give baby to Dad for 10 minutes and get a breath of fresh air.

- ❧ You will know if your baby is truly in distress.

- ❧ Eating well and keeping up your fluids is necessary for abundant breast-milk production.

- ❧ Take support and advice from those who have successfully breast-fed their own children.

- ❧ Breast feeding is not a medical event or experience; it is a natural process that takes some time and skill to master.

- ❧ After a couple of weeks, you'll feel like an old pro at it.

❧ SORE NIPPLES ☙

Whether you are a first-time mom or a champion nurser, you may experience sore nipples during the first few days of getting accustomed to nursing your baby. To prevent sore nipples, be sure that the baby is positioned well on your nipple, with a good mouthful, not just hanging on the edge of the nipple ("cliff-hanging"); avoid breast pads and tight bras, both of which keep moisture trapped near the nipple and lead to thrush; and allow your nipples to be exposed to air and sunlight for 20 minutes each day to keep them dry. If your baby has oral thrush, this must be treated, along with treating your nipples, as you will pass it back and forth to each other, and it will make breast feeding an extremely painful experience for you.

Here are some tips to soothe sore nipples:

- ❧ For cracked, dry, red nipples, regularly apply herbal salve made with comfrey root and calendula until your nipples become moisturized and heal. (Wipe off the salve before nursing—comfrey root is not safe for internal consumption by the baby.)

- ❧ Use cocoa butter, almond oil, vitamin E, or lanolin on your nipples. Some folks are allergic to lanolin, so discontinue its use if you notice a reaction. Wipe off any residue before you nurse your baby.

- ❧ Aloe vera gel applied to nipples brings cooling relief and helps heal cracks and cuts. It is intensely bitter, so rinse your nipples before nursing.

- ❧ Expose your nipples to fresh air and sunlight, or at least the latter, for 20 minutes a day. If cold or privacy is a problem, sunlight coming in through the window is adequate.

- ❧ If your nipples are painfully sore when you feed your baby, try nursing on one side for a day while you treat the other; then switch sides. This will not interfere with nursing and may give your nipples the needed time to heal.

TREATING THRUSH NATURALLY IN MOM AND BABY

A major cause of thrush, an infection with *Candida*, or yeast, in both Mom and baby, is the use of antibiotics during labor or after the birth. Thrush can also be picked up during a vaginal birth by a baby born to a mom with an active vaginal yeast infection, and this then is transmitted to the mom's nipples via the baby's mouth. Yeast thrives in warm, moist, dark environments. Typical medical treatment involves the use of antifungal drugs such as Nystatin, which should be reserved for extreme, intractable cases. The use of oral application of gentian violet is commonly recommended, but may be associated with oral cancer and thus is best avoided.

Treating Your Nipples

- ⁓ Wash your bras after daily use.
- ⁓ Dry bras at a high temperature setting or in the sun.
- ⁓ Avoid the use of breast pads and shields.
- ⁓ Expose your nipples to direct or indirect (through a window) sunlight for 20 minutes daily.
- ⁓ Go shirtless for 20 or more minutes daily to allow air to circulate to your nipples.
- ⁓ Use excellent hygiene, keeping nipples clean and dry.
- ⁓ Avoid eating foods high in sugar, as these contribute to yeast development.
- ⁓ Apply plain unsweetened yogurt or apple cider vinegar (2 tablespoons of vinegar to $1/2$ cup of water) to the nipples after each nursing.
- ⁓ Apply black walnut tincture to the breast four times daily. This stains, so be careful about clothing and bedding. Dilute tea tree *(Melaleuca)* tincture may be used topically as an alternative to black walnut.
- ⁓ For severe cases, apply a paste of aloe vera gel and goldenseal powder to the nipples after each nursing. Rinse off before you nurse as this paste is very bitter and not intended for consumption by your baby.
- ⁓ Use vitamin E oil or calendula oil on the nipples to heal cuts or sores.
- ⁓ Continue all treatments until the problem clears up.

Treating Thrush in the Baby

Thrush must also be treated in the baby to prevent it being passed back and forth between you. Nonmedical treatments can be effective, and are safer. For severe thrush, seek the care of your pediatrician.

- Swab the baby's mouth 4 times daily with a cotton swab dipped in black walnut tincture. *Caution:* do not substitute tea tree tincture. Do not replace the cotton swab into the bottle of tincture after it has been in the baby's mouth.

- Using your finger, swab the baby's mouth 4 times a day with plain, unsweetened yogurt, allowing the baby to swallow some. This promotes the growth of healthy flora, which control the growth of yeast.

❧ DIFFICULTY NURSING ☙

Many little difficulties can arise during the early stages of the breast-feeding relationship, including trouble getting the baby to latch on; the baby falling asleep as soon as she gets to your breast; the baby gagging or choking on mouthfuls of milk that come out uncontrollably fast; the baby becoming frustrated and screaming at the breast instead of nursing; and sore nipples. Any of these small concerns at the time may seem overwhelming to you; thus, it is incredibly important to have a supportive friend or guide who is experienced with breast feeding to help you understand and solve the problems.

There are few issues that arise, other than true medical problems, that will prevent a mother from successfully breast-feeding her baby provided she is determined and supported. Your partner needs to know in advance how important it is to you to breast-feed and should share your commitment—then his support will be fully behind you should you face challenges in the early days of nursing, or even later on in the breast-feeding relationship.

❧ INSUFFICIENT BREAST MILK ☙

Most women can and do produce enough breast milk to amply and abundantly feed their babies. Unless you have a pituitary or other hormonal problem, suffer from certain specific medical problems, or have had breast surgery (reduction and augmentation can interfere with the ability to breast-feed, although neither definitively interferes with nursing), it is unlikely your body will have difficulty producing adequate milk. Good indicators that your baby is getting enough milk include six to eight wet diapers per day (though there may normally be significantly fewer in the first 48 hours after birth—check with your pediatrician to make sure) and the baby making swallowing sounds while nursing. Eventually, weight gain is another sign. If you don't see milk dribbling out of your baby's mouth after each feeding, or don't see milk pouring out of your breasts, and even if you're unable to express milk, this doesn't mean you don't have adequate breast milk. Signs that should concern you and which may indicate dehydration or inadequate nutrition include dry mucous membranes in the baby's mouth, lethargy in the baby, significant weight loss, and a sunken fontanel (on the top of the baby's head). Should you observe these signs, contact your pediatrician immediately.

Having adequate milk and a good let-down or "milk ejection" reflex are two entirely different issues. In order for the baby to get your milk, the milk ducts must experience a contractile wave triggered by a hormone produced in your brain. This allows your body to release the breast milk. This physiologic action is known as the let-down reflex, and may be pronounced in some women and barely noticeable in others. Women who experience a pronounced sensation describe it as tingling or feeling like little shards of crystals are moving through their ducts. After several weeks, it becomes a barely noticeable sensation. The let-down reflex can be inhibited by stress and anxiety; therefore, it is important that you feel good about breast-feeding your baby for your experience to be successful and satisfying. Inhibition about nursing in public, discomfort with nursing a baby of the opposite sex (or same sex), and other psychological or emotional issues regarding breast feeding need to be addressed openly and resolved.

Midwives and wise women have long used herbs to ensure a plentiful supply of breast milk. Although drinking adequate amounts of water and eating well should be sufficient, many of these herbs promote relaxation in the mother and can encourage let-down while improving the nutritional quality of the milk and preventing colic in your baby. Below are some of my favorite herbs and milk-friendly herbal tea recipes, safe for baby and Mom.

❧ Mother's Milk Tea Blend

This is a tasty and soothing blend of herbs for new moms, but you may find yourself drinking it as a comfort tea for years to come. Children love it, too.

    1 ounce dried chamomile flowers
    1 ounce dried catnip

$^1/_4$ ounce fennel seeds

$^1/_8$ ounce dried lavender flowers

Combine all the herbs. Put 1 tablespoon of the mix in a cup and fill with boiling water. Cover the cup and let steep for 10 minutes. Strain and drink plain or slightly sweetened.

Dose: 1–3 cups daily

 Nourishment Tea

A refreshing green and slightly minty tea, this is rich in trace minerals and excellent for enriching the quality and quantity of your breast milk. Your kids, too, are bound to like this one.

1 ounce dried nettle leaf

1 ounce red raspberry leaves

$^1/_2$ ounce alfalfa leaf

$^1/_2$ ounce red clover blossoms

$^1/_2$ ounce rose hips

$^1/_4$–$^1/_2$ ounce spearmint leaf (to taste)

Combine all the herbs. Steep 4 tablespoons per quart of boiling water for 30 minutes. Strain, then drink plain or slightly sweetened. Makes an excellent hot or cool beverage and is delicious with squeezed lemon.

Dose: Up to 4 cups daily

Beer is an old wives' brew for increasing milk supply. It's high in calories, which helps increase the amount of milk you produce, and the hops and the alcohol encourage you to relax. This helps the let-down. Nonalcoholic beers provide some of the same benefits as their alcohol-containing cousins, without your having to pass alcohol on to the baby via your breast milk.

❧ BREAST-FEEDING SUPPORT ☙ IN THE DAYS AFTER BIRTH

Breast-feeding support and encouragement are best gained from those who have successfully breast-fed their own babies. There are tips, tricks, and skills— as well as confidence—that can be learned only from direct experience. In a society where breast feeding is the norm, your own mother would be supportive and helpful. In the United States, where breast feeding has been uncommon for the past few generations, grandmothers themselves are apt to have bottle-fed and thus are inexperienced with breast feeding. They therefore may be unable to help the new mother successfully establish breast feeding. Furthermore, they may not realize that to establish a successful breast-feeding relationship, the mother must be the one who primarily holds and comforts the baby for the first few days after birth. Many new grandmothers are all too inclined to try to hold and comfort baby so Mom can rest, when what really needs to happen is that they take care of everything else—such as food, housework, and older children—so Mom can hold baby and both can rest.

La Leche League, an international organization started by mothers who wanted to breast-feed their babies, is dedicated to supporting, educating, and encouraging breast-feeding mothers, with chapters in cities and towns all over the world. There is no charge to contact La Leche League for information, and it is a simple matter to find a local group. Call 1-800-LA-LECHE for more information.

BREAST MILK IS BEST

The benefits of breast feeding are innumerable. Researchers are just beginning to recognize the increased immune response and enhanced intellectual development in breast-fed babies. Breast-fed babies in general are healthier, have higher IQ scores; are less likely to be obese as adults; have a decreased risk of childhood and adult-onset diabetes; receive higher-quality nutrients including essential fatty acids; and have better eyesight, hearing, teeth, and respiratory functioning than those not breast-fed. Furthermore, they will have healthier hearts, lower cholesterol, and better digestion. And the benefits in most of these areas increase with the length of breast feeding. If we place our trust in our bodies and in nature, then it is logical to assume that our breasts produce milk after we give birth for important reasons.

The trend in bottle-feeding in the past few generations is directly linked to economic motives from both the public and the private sectors. Prior to World War II, babies were almost always breast-fed. But during the war, so many men had to leave the workforce to join the Army that women were required to take their place in order to keep the economy functioning and to serve the war effort. As women left the home, bottle-feeding became more common. Around the same time, the newly founded bottle-feeding industry, along with physicians, promoted the notion that babies could not grow adequately on breast milk. My husband's grandmother often told me the story of how her doctor "made her" weigh her son (my father-in-law) before breast-feeding him, then again immediately after he nursed. If he did not gain a certain number of ounces in a feeding, she was to supplement him with formula. Of course, with such a routine and with such doubt cast over her ability to nourish her son at her breast, nursing did not last long. This is not an uncommon story.

Since World War II, billions of dollars have been made in the production of formula and other feeding paraphernalia—"the necessities of motherhood"—and the industry continues to grow. Hospitals receive thousands of dollars from formula makers for the endorsement of their brands. We have been brainwashed into believing that food from a cow, put into a can and bought in a store, is better for our babies than is the milk from our own breasts, which is free!

❧ IF YOU AREN'T BREAST-FEEDING ☙

Breast feeding is the best choice for you if that is what you want to do. Although there is no doubt that it provides the optimal nutrition for your baby, it may not be right for everyone, and a very small number of you, for a variety of medical or personal reasons, might not be able to breast-feed.

If you have chosen not to nurse, your midwife or pediatrician can help you choose the best formula for your baby. There are several considerations— for example, whether to use a dairy- or a soy-based product. Some parents have turned to soy or rice milk as a formula substitute. *These are not adequate or safe baby foods.* If you choose to give your baby formula, use a product that is designed to be baby formula, and preferably one that is approved by the FDA for that purpose.

Goat's milk, when properly fortified for a newborn's needs, could be a satisfactory substitute. Speak to your pediatrician about this possibility.

To dry up your breast milk naturally, drink 2 to 3 cups of sage *(Salvia officinalis)* tea daily. To prepare: Steep 1 heaping teaspoon of dried or 2 teaspoons of fresh sage leaf in 1 cup of boiling water, covered, for 10 minutes. Strain, sweeten lightly with honey, and drink.

Breast-feeding is best, but it is not the only way to ensure an emotionally close relationship with your child. Always hold your baby while bottle-feeding, and express your love fully. This love will provide enormous emotional security, psychological wellness, and physical comfort to your baby.

COMPARISON OF BREAST FEEDING AND FORMULA FEEDING

Concern	Breast Feeding	Formula Feeding
Nutrients	Ideal food for human babies; composition changes to meet their needs as they grow.	Modeled after but not the same as human milk. Composition doesn't change over time. Must be prepared carefully to supply proper nutrition and can become contaminated.
Quantity	Underfeeding and dehydration can be a problem for newborns if mother is not knowledgeable about breast-feeding and infant-feeding needs or signs of malnutrition.	Overfeeding is a risk and may be associated with childhood and adult overweight and obesity.
Immunity	Immune factors in the mother are conferred to the baby and are now known to provide long-lasting and significant immunity to the baby well after the breast-feeding relationship has been discontinued.	There are no immune factors in formula.
Allergies	Babies are rarely allergic to breast milk, and breast-feeding reduces the risk of developing food allergies.	Babies may be sensitive to soy or dairy components of infant formula; formula fed babies are more likely to develop food allergies.
Health risks	Environmental contaminants, medications, illicit drugs, and certain diseases (hepatitis, HIV) can be transmitted from mother to baby via breast milk.	Food-based contaminants can be passed to the baby via formula, but the composition of the formula is not affected by the mother's health or substance intake.
Environmental risks	Breast milk is sterile; pumped milk can become contaminated if not stored correctly. Lower environmental impact as no manufacturing and packaging are required.	Bacterial contamination is a risk from improperly stored or prepared formula.

Concern	Breast Feeding	Formula Feeding
Convenience	Always available, no preparation or cleanup. Mother must be available to feed baby or pump and store milk.	More preparation and cleanup but feeding responsibility can be shared by others.
Ease for baby	Sucking takes more effort but provides stronger facial muscle development necessary for speech.	Easier for sick or weak babies to obtain food.
Physical and Psychological Benefits	Promotes healthy return of the uterus to prepregnant size; may be more psychologically and emotionally satisfying to mother and baby.	Little physical benefit to mother or baby; allows mother to be more independent of baby.
Costs	No costs but the mother must be well nourished.	More expensive than breast feeding.

Adapted from *Nutrition: Science and Applications*, Smolin and Grosvenor

❧ REFLECTING ON YOUR BIRTH ☙

Birth is a once-in-a-lifetime experience that leaves an indelible imprint on your psyche. Indeed, while mothers might forget various details of their childrearing experience, most women retain the details of each child's birth with remarkable vividness. However, time can fade some of these details; therefore, I encourage women to create a birth story in the first week after each baby is born, recording the labor and birth chronologically. This is also a wonderful record to keep for your son or daughter, who years later might wonder what his or her own birth was like. One possibility is to create a small gift book for your child, with photos of you pregnant, newborn pictures, your birth story, and other memorabilia that reminds you of the experience or of the time when you were pregnant. Such a gift is destined to be a family heirloom for many generations.

❧ A DIFFICULT BIRTH ☙

During pregnancy you may have built up strong expectations of how your birth will be. Your actual birth experience, however, may be quite different from your ideals. Perhaps you intended to have a home birth or birthing center birth but had to go to the hospital; perhaps your partner was not as involved or supportive as you imagined he would be; perhaps you prepared for an unmedicated birth but chose to have an epidural; perhaps the birth culminated in an emergency cesarean section. Of course, you are undoubtedly grateful that you and your baby are well, but you may still feel significant disappointment in yourself, your caregivers, your partner, even some resentment toward the baby. It is very important to review the details of the birth with honesty and self-reflection, and not hold back on the tears, anger, or disappointment.

Time and perspective will help you understand more deeply what you felt hurt or disappointed about, but raw feelings after the birth can easily become suppressed emotions if they are not in some way addressed or processed. Writing down these feelings can provide both relief and a framework for constructive action in order to come to peace with or heal the situation about which you feel unresolved. Talking to an understanding friend can sometimes be very helpful, as can speaking to or expressing in writing your feelings to your care provider, support people, or partner. Although you cannot always get the responses you hope for, you can prevent yourself from having pent-up feelings during a time when your energy should focus on healing and nourishing.

❧ EMOTIONAL HIGHS AND LOWS ❧

The days after birth are a time of mercurial emotions—your feelings change from moment to moment, along with your quickly fluctuating hormones and your rapidly shifting sense of identity. Understanding the volatile and capricious nature of postpartum emotions in advance can help you recognize and face them when they happen to you. If your birth was not how you hoped it would be, particularly if trauma was involved, your emotions are even more likely to swing from one extreme to the other. As discussed earlier, it is critically important that you find a way to express and process your feelings about your birth experience, and anything else that might be troubling you at this time. However, some of the fluctuating nature of your emotions is hormonal, and can be balanced with excellent diet and adequate rest and fluids. Herbal preparations can be useful for helping the hormones to adjust, as well as to soothe jangled nerves. The following recipes are highly recommend for use during the early postpartum, may be continued for months after birth, and are considered safe for use while breast-feeding. Consider having some of these on hand prior to birth so you don't have to send anyone on a special mission to find them later.

Keeping-Your-Balance Blend

This personal formula for emotional well-being is a modified version of Women's Balancing Blend, created by Rosemary Gladstar Slick. You can prepare it at home.

> $^1/_2$ ounce chamomile flowers
> $^1/_2$ ounce chrysanthemum flowers
> $^1/_2$ ounce nettles
> $^1/_2$ ounce oatstraw
> $^1/_2$ ounce peppermint
> $^1/_2$ ounce red raspberry leaves
> $^1/_2$ ounce strawberry leaves
> $^1/_4$ ounce dandelion leaves
> $^1/_4$ ounce gingerroot
> $^1/_4$ ounce rose petals

In a medium bowl, blend all the herbs. Steep 1 tablespoon of the blend in 1 cup of boiling water for 20 minutes, or use 1 handful per quart jar of water. *Dose:* Drink up to 6 cups a day, plain or sweetened. It's delicious!

Catnip and Motherwort Combination

This excellent combination helps take the rough edges off your emotions, particularly if you're weeping a lot or are experiencing irritability. It supports breast-milk production, promotes rest, and supports uterine tone, so is an all-around boon for you during this time.

Prepare as for Keeping-Your-Balance Blend.

Dose: The dose for emotional swings is 1 teaspoon every 2 to 4 hours, as needed. This can be maintained for several weeks at a time.

Use Mother's Milk Tea Blend (see page 107) freely during this time to maintain relaxation, reduce stress, and keep the emotions as balanced as possible. Remember, though, emotions are the doorway into our soul. Try not to repress or ignore them. Keep a journal or find another means to express yourself, and if your emotions are persistently extreme, find a trusted friend or professional to talk to.

BODY TONICS

You may take herbs internally in the first few days after birth to promote recovery and strength. Several recommended specifics are partridgeberry, a uterine tonic (take 1 teaspoon 2 or 3 times daily); motherwort, a uterine tonic and nervine (1 teaspoon 2 or 3 times daily); gotu kola, which aids in the repair of connective tissue damage (use as a tea, 2 cups daily, or a tincture, $^1/_2$ to 1 teaspoon twice daily); shepherd's purse (tea or tincture, as for gotu kola), which allays bleeding; and nettles (infusion of 1 ounce of herb per quart of boiling water, steeped 1 hour), which replenishes nutrients and helps balance blood sugar. Combine into a tincture blend, to be taken in a dose of 1 teaspoon 3 times daily, or add individual tinctures to other teas. Continue for the first 5 days postpartum.

In Chinese medicine, the placenta is traditionally made into a medicine to be taken by the mother in the days postnatally. Bob Flaws, in his book *The Path of Pregnancy*, writes: "Postpartum discharge and tonification can be facilitated through the use of the placenta. . . . The placenta is full of hormones and other biologically powerful substances. It is very potent and powerful medicine and should not be wasted."

Although taking the placenta as medicine may not be everyone's cup of tea, many of my clients over the years have done this and found it very tonifying. The following instructions allow you to dry and preserve the placenta as a powder, which, kept in a dark, cool environment, will keep for years. However, the recommendation is to take it during the first week or 10 days postpartum until it is entirely used up.

 Placenta Power
1 slice (1 inch) fresh gingerroot
$^1/_4$ slice fresh lemon
$^1/_2$ ounce tienchi ginseng (optional)

Preheat the oven to 300°F. Clean the placenta thoroughly of all blood and clots within a few hours of the birth. Strip away the membranes and cord with a sharp knife. Place the placenta on a metal steamer rack in a pot filled with 1 to 2 inches of water. On top of the placenta, place the gingerroot and lemon. Cover the pot and steam for 20 minutes. Turn off heat, turn the placenta over, and repeat the process on the other side.

Next, remove the ginger and lemon and slice the placenta into thin strips. Place on a baking tray and bake until completely dry, about 2 hours. Allow to cool to room temperature for several hours, then place all the slices in a blender and pulverize to a coarse powder. Place in "00"-sized capsules.

If the mother is weak, buy steamed tienchi ginseng, 40 grams (1¹/₂ ounces) in powder form and add it to the placenta powder before encapsulating. This is more fortifying.
Dose: Take 2 capsules, three times daily

❧   EXERCISE   ☙

You'll have plenty of time to regain the physical shape you lost during the pregnancy; the first week after birth is not a time to rejoin an aerobics—or even yoga—class. During the first couple of days, just take it easy and continue pelvic-floor (Kegel) exercises from pregnancy to reinforce the tone of your pelvic floor. Start with a few repetitions and work your way up to 100 a day. This is a healthy habit for a lifetime, preventing later problems with pelvic organ prolapse, which is fairly common. You can also begin to do gentle side-lying leg lifts and alternating leg lifts lying on your back (see illustrations on page 222).

During the first 2 weeks, I encourage new moms not to lift anything heavier than the baby, and to let the amount they bleed indicate reasonable activity level. Too much activity will cause heavy bleeding and is a good gauge of whether you are overexerting yourself. The next chapter will provide you with tips on exercising in the first 6 weeks after birth.

❧   SEX AFTER BIRTH   ☙

For a lot of women who have just given birth, sex during the first week—or even months—after birth is the farthest thing from their minds. There are those women and men alike who find birth and breast feeding very sexy. Although it is not necessarily unsafe to have sex in the first week after a healthy vaginal birth with no interventions, midwives and obstetricians generally recommend waiting a couple of weeks, or until the bleeding has begun to substantially subside. If you had an episiotomy or cesarean, it is preferable to wait for several weeks for your wounds to heal. Intimacy can be achieved in many ways, and it may be your body's natural instinct or response to the experience of birth to be uninterested in sex.

Bear in mind that your fertility can return even in the first few weeks after birth. Being postpartum, even if you are breast-feeding, is no guarantee of pregnancy prevention. When you do resume sexual intimacy, be sure to use contraception. The next chapters will discuss sexuality in the months after birth.

❧ YOUR HEALTHY NEWBORN ❧

This book is written specifically for and about the needs of new mothers, but it is clear that the focus of a new mother is largely her baby. Therefore, this book would be incomplete without some discussion of what you can expect from your baby in the first days after birth. For a more thorough discussion of the needs of newborns and young children, I encourage you to read my book *Naturally Healthy Babies and Children,* and to refer to the Further Reading section of that book and to the bibliography in this one.

Here let's look at some basic information about what you can expect from a healthy newborn. You'll learn about the baby's vital signs, how to interpret your baby's "language," and how to recognize when your baby is ill.

Before addressing the topic of newborn care, I want to acknowledge again the important connection between the health of the mother and that of her baby. A well-nourished mother has the most likelihood of birthing a healthy baby. Strong babies, likewise, have the most resilience. Habits such as cigarette smoking and drug use during pregnancy have a proven link with prenatal, birth, and childhood health problems. There is a greater possibility of premature birth, low birth weight, developmental anomalies, and even respiratory problems in toddlers. Babies born with an adequate birth weight (over $6\frac{1}{2}$ pounds) to mothers in good health are at the least risk for such problems.

In the same way that a healthy pregnant mother will usually have a healthy baby, health in a breast-feeding baby is directly related to the mom's well-being. Breast feeding fortifies children against illness, but a woman must be in good health if she is going to provide nourishing milk to her child. Similarly, when the baby is sick, working with the nursing mother's diet and giving herbal remedies directly to the mother will benefit the baby. In the pediatric philosophy of traditional Chinese medicine, the main approach to restoring health to an ill breast-feeding baby is to treat the mother.

Even when women don't breast-feed, their health affects their babies. If a mother doesn't take care of herself, she is more likely to become ill or exhausted. She will then be exposing the baby to her illness or, at the least, may be too tired to provide the baby with the care he needs. This is true of the father as well. The responsibility parents have may seem daunting, but we can choose to take pride in the great influence we have on our children through the examples we set. We can, from the start, influence them in a direction that teaches the correlation between the actions we take and how they affect our wellness, and also how we affect others.

YOUR BABY'S APPEARANCE

Shortly after birth, most babies have a slightly ruddy appearance, which gradually fades to a nice natural skin color over the first couple of days. For the first 24 hours, some babies have bluish hands and feet, which is usually normal, though you should mention it to your midwife or healthcare provider.

When the baby comes through the birth canal, the bones of the head overlap to a greater or lesser degree, depending on the tightness of the fit and the length of time spent in the canal. This normal physiological process, known as molding, gives some babies a "cone-head" appearance. After the first day the baby's head has usually assumed a nice round shape. Likewise, if the nose was pressed a bit flat at birth, it begins to perk up in the first postpartum days.

Newborns have an incredible purity about them, down to the smallest details of their beings. Their scent is indescribably fresh and sweet (I always think of the scent of the air after a spring thundershower). Their eyes open wide and drink in all that they see with a receptive mind and nonjudgmental heart, and babies speak a million words without a sound. Their tiny fingers grasp and hold with firmness. If you spend an extra minute, you can feel yourself melt into oneness with that child. Just to be in the presence of a newborn is magical. Their stillness when sleeping brings peace to our busy minds as nothing else can.

Take the time to gaze into your baby's eyes, look at her toes, hold his hand, nuzzle her head, and fill yourself with his scent. You will begin a relationship that enables you to know your child deeply and closely, and this relationship will be the best guide to your child's health that you can ever have.

Regularly checking your baby's "vital signs" is unnecessary (except for temperature, which your midwife may want you to check a few times daily for the first few days after birth). But if you have any concerns about your baby's well-being, there are a few basics to consider.

TEMPERATURE

Every baby has his own rhythms and preferences, but some things are pretty standard. A newborn's temperature measured rectally averages 98.6 degrees F (37 degrees C). An easy, less invasive alternative to rectal measurement is to put the tip of the thermometer in the baby's armpit and snuggle the baby's arm down against his side for 5 minutes. This is called the axillary temperature and is typically one degree lower than rectal measurement (so 97.6 degrees is normal). Forehead and other types of thermometers may also be used, following the directions on their packages.

Any newborn with an elevated temperature needs close attention, though it may still be considered normal at 99 degrees F for the first 24 hours. Most often, the baby is overdressed or slightly dehydrated. Remove blankets and keep the baby in just a diaper and T-shirt if the room is warm. Check the baby's temperature again after 15 minutes. If it is still elevated, sponge the baby's wrists, feet, and forehead with tepid water (not cold!), and give the baby the breast or a bit of boiled water (cooled to room temperature) by eyedropper, providing liquid to drink until he'll take no more. If after an hour the temperature is still above normal, or if the baby shows signs of illness (see the end of this chapter), seek an experienced midwife or a physician immediately.

Babies need to be kept warm, not swelteringly hot. By touching the skin you can tell if your baby is too warm or cold. Generally, the feet and hands should feel comfortably warm but slightly cooler than the chest and back. If the baby's hands feel quite warm, she may be overdressed or running a fever. Adjust the child's clothing and the room temperature accordingly; then recheck the baby's temperature.

A baby who looks white or mottled or who has blue hands or feet may be chilled. A baby who appears ruddy may be too hot. These color changes may also indicate serious health concerns, so consult your care provider if adjusting clothing and room temperature doesn't solve the problem.

BREATHING

A baby's breathing is often irregular, possibly with occasional lapses for up to 12 seconds. Babies sometimes may also take little gulps of air. However, a baby's breathing should be effortless. There should be no grunting or wheezing sounds, and the chest should not heave. If your baby stops breathing for longer than 12 seconds, turns blue, or exhibits any of the signs of respiratory distress just mentioned, get immediate help. Your baby could have an infection or another problem that needs attention.

The normal breathing rate is 30 to 40 breaths per minute. Sometimes the respiratory rate is up to 60 breaths a minute on the first day after birth. To compute the breathing rate, just listen closely and count how many breaths your baby takes in 60 seconds (use a watch or clock with a second hand as you count).

Babies commonly sneeze in the first couple of days after birth; this is how they clear their breathing passages. A tiny bit of rattling mucus in the nose will clear itself out with sneezes. Healthy newborns, however, do not have runny noses.

HEARTBEAT

To check your baby's heart rate, put your fingers or ear over her heart and count the beats for 1 minute. A healthy baby's heart rate averages 110 to 150 beats each minute, fluctuating according to sleeping, nursing, and movement. A healthy baby may have a sleeping heart rate as low as 80 beats per minute. A baby whose heartbeat is well above or below this range may have a health problem, so speak with your midwife or physician promptly.

SLEEPING

Each newborn sleeps a varying amount depending on personality. Some newborns take naps for hours at a time; others take short, frequent naps. Babies commonly and normally fall asleep soon after being put to the breast. Many times they will continue to nurse during a nap.

There really is no rule about how much sleep is acceptable for newborns, but babies should have some alert and bright-eyed times each day and should be eager to nurse even if they doze while doing so. Physicians generally recommend babies not be allowed to sleep more than 4 hours at a time during the day, for fear they won't eat often enough if they sleep too much. In practice, I've found that babies usually wake to nurse or eat within this time frame. If your baby is not showing signs of jaundice, infection, or general lethargy (see "Signs of Illness in the Newborn," page 123), there is no harm in longer naps.

Much to the chagrin of their parents, some babies sleep very little. For unknown reasons, they take few naps or very short naps, keeping their parents on call most of the day. Most babies will sleep a considerable amount during the first few days or even weeks after the birth; however, there are newborns who quickly kick the nap habit and want to nurse (or eat) and be held nearly all day. Fortunately, these babies often sleep well at night, though not always.

If you have such a baby, try to arrange for time each day, particularly in the first few months after the birth, when you can take a shower, nap, enjoy a decent meal, or replenish yourself in any way you need to in order to maintain your health (and sanity!). Be sure to relax when the baby does nap, and get to sleep early at night. Full-time parenting of a child who doesn't sleep much, no matter how much you adore him, can quickly become draining. If you take good care of yourself, you will have more energy for your high-maintenance baby. Eventually your baby will learn to sleep through the night, but for the time being, develop your support system so you don't burn out. And "wearing" your baby in a sling or backpack during the day gives you time with your hands free, simultaneously keeping baby happily occupied.

EATING

Some babies take a little while after birth to start nursing—even a few hours or more. How much a baby nurses will vary, but it is generally felt that a newborn should nurse at least every 3 to 4 hours. (I usually don't wake my babies just to nurse if they nurse with enthusiasm when they wake on their own.) Most newborns nurse more often than that. If your baby refuses your breast but has no health problems, be patient but persistent in order to establish nursing. Given this, breast feeding will usually begin within the first 24 hours. If not, seek the support of a La Leche League leader, a lactation consultant, or a healthcare worker such as your midwife, who can teach you how to express and feed the baby your milk via another route until he begins to suckle. This is necessary to prevent the baby from becoming dehydrated or hypoglycemic.

A listless, lethargic baby who does not want to nurse much is probably not feeling well and may have a condition that requires attention.

It is fine to offer your breast to baby whenever she cries or if you think she may be hungry. A baby will suckle only if she wants to; she'll push away your nipple with her lips if she doesn't want to nurse.

Spitting up is common and is usually just some overflow regurgitated from the stomach. To cut down on spitting up, feed your baby in a calm environment, and hold the baby firmly and lovingly, without jiggling and bouncing. A baby with projectile vomiting (long-distance, forceful vomiting) needs medical attention. If after you nurse you pick up your little one with your hands around his belly, forcing his food back up, don't worry; that is not projectile vomiting.

Each baby has his own nursing style. Some nurse heartily for 2-hour stretches; others take sips here and there. The frequency and amount of elimination is a good indication of whether your baby is eating enough, as is weight gain. Newborns begin to visibly fill out in the first weeks after birth.

ELIMINATION

A baby should urinate and have a bowel movement at least once in the first 24 hours after birth. After your milk comes in, the baby will usually wet a minimum of six diapers a day. For the first couple of days after birth, the baby's stools will be black and tarlike. These stools are called *meconium* and are what was in your baby's intestines before birth. After the first few days, the poops turn a golden brown and have a loose consistency. Babies have unique bowel habits ranging anywhere from a few a day to a few over a couple of days. If your baby is not having a bowel movement at least every two days, look at your diet to rule out anything that could be constipating the baby. Common causes are dairy foods, peanut butter, wheat, and red meat.

CRYING

It's a fact of life that even the happiest babies sometimes cry, for one simple reason: Crying is their language. A newborn cannot simply say, "My diaper is wet—will you please change it?" If you don't notice that your baby needs a diaper change, then after a while he must inform you. Crying is probably the technique he'll use.

Some babies are more patient than others, and some parents are so incredibly attentive that their babies rarely cry. Breast-fed babies may actually cry less often than their bottle-fed counterparts because the relationship between mother and child tends to be very intimate, and the moms quickly learn to respond to their babies' subtle messages. But even breast-fed babies fuss and cry. All children teethe, get overtired, suffer an occasional ache or fright, or have a reason to become inconsolable at some point before they go off to college.

Because a fussy baby can be trying on our patience, our task is to learn to comfort our kids when possible or even to let them cry for a bit if necessary without taking their unhappiness personally and without become so frustrated that we lash out at them. If you are holding your beautiful baby peacefully asleep in your arms at this moment, the idea of being irritated at such an angel may seem hard to imagine, but someday at 4 in the morning, pacing with a teething baby, perhaps you'll remember this page. The most common reason parents in child-abuse cases give for battering a baby is that the baby just wouldn't stop crying. There is, of course, absolutely no excuse for abusing a child. You must learn how to cope.

If your baby is fussy, irritable, or even screaming, here are some basic steps you can take to comfort him without losing your cool. First, carefully look over your baby from head to toe to be certain that nothing is causing physical discomfort. Even a hair that has become tightly wound around a finger or toe can cause extreme pain, as well as endanger the circulation of that body part. Another possibility is that your baby has colic (see chapter 7). If the baby doesn't seem to have any physical injuries, has no fever, normally does not get colic, and is fed, has a dry diaper, and isn't too hot or too cold, try to play with or rock him. Of course, if the baby is hurt or sick, you need to take the steps appropriate for that situation.

If the baby is fine but fussy despite your efforts to offer comfort, and you are becoming irritated or exhausted, put the baby down somewhere safe and get some fresh air or go to a quiet place in your house for just a few minutes or for as long as you need to gather your composure. If you're harried, the baby will perceive this through your body language (smell, muscular tension, irritable behavior) and will resist settling down. When you feel at peace, return to your baby and try again to offer comfort. Don't hesitate to enlist your spouse, or call a relative, friend, or even a neighbor if you are a single parent and need support. "Wearing" your baby in a sling while you go about your business will give baby a sense of closeness to you while allowing her to be gently rocked by the movement of your body. You'll feel less frustrated, and your baby is likely to drop off to sleep.

❧ SIGNS OF ILLNESS ☙ IN THE NEWBORN

Any baby who "just doesn't seem well" to the parents, particularly to the mom, should be evaluated by an experienced healthcare practitioner. Parents often have a keen sense of whether their children are well or ill.

WHEN TO SEEK MEDICAL CARE

Some signs of illness requiring the attention of a healthcare practitioner include: not wanting to nurse or eat; abnormal temperature; irritability combined with any of these signs; jaundice combined with any of these signs; bulging anterior fontanel (soft spot on baby's head); very stiff or floppy body; baby "just doesn't seem well."

If the baby is ill, consult with your midwife or physician to discuss the best approach for healing. When you determine the cause of the problem, you can refer to the next chapter for appropriate treatment possibilities. No matter where or how you choose to heal your baby, your love and constant presence are the most important medicine. Talk to, touch, nurse, cuddle, and reassure your newborn.

❧ BABIES IN NEED OF ❧ SPECIAL CARE

It is beyond the scope of this book to provide information on caring for babies with congenital or severe health problems, but it is important to me that their parents not feel left out of this discussion, as they will certainly have special needs as well. If your baby was born "different" from what you'd hoped or expected, please know that many support groups and loving people care deeply about children and can help you accept and learn to care for your child fully. Cascade Health Care Products has a parenting catalog, *Imprints*, that contains a fine selection of reading materials and videos on dealing with pregnancy loss and "special babies." Midwives can frequently help you locate resources in your community.

Should your baby require medical care, you can usually stay with him. Most hospitals are now supportive of breast feeding and sometimes even give babies their mothers' milk through tubes if nursing by mouth is impossible. Spending time with your baby adds to the chances of his quick recovery, particularly in the case of prematurity. Babies held and touched often are known to recover health and gain weight faster than those receiving minimal contact. If your baby is terminally ill, the contact you have will give you cherished memories to draw on in the years to come; and while the experience of illness or loss of a child is incredibly painful, those memories will help you, in time, to feel a sense of completion with the experience.

❧ GETTING ENOUGH REST ❧

It cannot be overemphasized: Rest as much as you possibly can during the first couple of weeks postpartum. It is particularly important to nap when the baby naps rather than give in to the temptation to pick up around the house, do errands, or catch up on other responsibilities. There will be time for all of that in a few weeks. If you have older children, nap while they're in school or ask a relative or a friend to help out with them for an hour or two each day. Get over feeling guilty for resting or lying around doing nothing but taking care of the baby. Put a sign on the door of your house that says DO NOT DISTURB: NEW MOM AND BABY RESTING. Let your answering machine screen calls for you, and return only the ones that are essential. I once received wise advice from a mother of five: Keep your pajamas on for the first week—once you get back into your regular clothes, you get back into your regular life. Consider purchasing a few special nightgowns (make sure you can breast-feed in them) for the first week after birth.

Remaining adequately rested will help keep your emotions level and allow you to have more energy for the baby and the rest of your family. This is definitely not the time to try to be a superwoman. This is the time to honor the recuperative needs of your body. It is also a sacred time when you can indulge in immersing yourself in getting to know your new little life companion without constant distraction. Allow yourself to enjoy this time. Bask in the nourishment of others. Sleep and lounge. Take baths. Eat well. If you're having difficulty resting because you're so excited, take Mother's Milk Tea Blend (see page 107), up to 4 cups daily, to promote relaxation.

Signs that you are not resting adequately include increased vaginal bleeding—particularly if it had already begun to subside—breast duct inflammation, fatigue, irritability, and colds. If you experience any of these signs or symptoms, increase rest time, stay off your feet more, and improve your nutritional intake. See your midwife or doctor if bleeding is persistent, or if you have any signs of infection.

❧ VISITORS, VISITORS, ❧ AND MORE VISITORS

Everybody loves to see a baby, and what parent doesn't want to show off her new little one. Indeed, babies bring a smile to just about anyone's face. Unfortunately, for new moms, too many visitors can bring about unnecessary exhaustion. Even talking on the phone in a prolonged conversation can be draining. The postpartum is a time for you to be preserving and pulling energy into yourself, not giving it out to family and friends. Others should be nurturing you.

After our babies were born, we put a nicely decorated note on our door to deter unsolicited visitors and remind welcome guests that we had unique needs at that time. Consider posting a note on your door such as the one below, and leave a message on your answering machine reminding people that you want to see them but you must keep visitors to a minimum and visits brief during the first 2 weeks after the birth.

> *Welcome, Visitors.*
>   *Please note that new moms and babies need lots of rest and quiet. We ask you to keep visits quiet and no longer than 15 minutes if you are just coming to peek at the baby.*
>   *If you are planning to stay longer, please be prepared to play with our older children, throw in a load of laundry, or get a meal started.*
>   *Thanks for your patience and understanding.*

⅔ᴗ NEW MAMA NUTRITION ᴄ⅘

Paying attention to nutrition during pregnancy can be time-consuming and exhausting, as you try to eat carefully to ensure your baby's proper growth and development. Many women find this awesome responsibility almost overwhelming and are relieved when pregnancy is over and they can go back to eating "normally." However, nutrition during breast-feeding is also important. William and Martha Sears, in *The Breastfeeding Book*, sum up nutrition and breast feeding this way:

> During lactation, as during pregnancy, your body nourishes your baby's body. Just as your blood carried the nutrients your baby needed to grow and develop in the womb, your milk furnishes all the nutrients your baby needs after birth. Mothers over the world make good-quality milk for their babies, many of them with less than adequate diets for themselves. . . . A mother's body guards valuable nutrients during pregnancy and lactation. Calcium, for example, is absorbed more efficiently and less is excreted. There's no need to obsess about having to eat "just right" while breastfeeding. In a nutshell, good nutrition while breastfeeding means eating foods that are good for you—and a bit more than you would normally consume.

During the first few days postpartum you have unique considerations. First of all, many women are nervous about having a bowel movement soon after birth. Avoiding constipation and difficult elimination is the key to healthy digestion. Eat plenty of fruits and vegetables, drink ample quantities of water, and keep away from hard-to-digest foods such as peanut butter, dairy products, and red meat (with the exception of red meat cooked in stews). Raisin bran muffins made with blackstrap molasses are a natural laxative, as are stewed or soaked prunes. Chapter 6 addresses nutrition and breast feeding extensively.

Although pregnancy is a natural process, it still puts strain on your body. The body also needs to expend energy for healing after birth, and if there has been significant blood loss, iron and other nutrients must be replaced. Furthermore, breast-milk production, believe it or not, requires even greater caloric intake than does pregnancy. This is because you are continuing to provide primary nourishment for a rapidly growing baby undergoing not only enormous physical development, but also tremendous brain development in the first 6 months after birth.

Traditional foods for women in the immediate postpartum period are amazingly similar cross-culturally. Foods typically include soups or stews with grains (for example, barley stew); meat and vegetable soups (for example, chicken soup); plenty of eggs, chicken, and grains; and starchy vegetables (sweet potatoes, winter squash). Fruits in season may be encouraged as well. Cooked raisins and jujube dates feature prominently in the dietary recommendations for Chinese women who have recently given birth. Such foods nourish the blood, while the protein in them helps with the speedy and effective repair and replenishment of body tissue.

Avoid foods that might irritate the breast-feeding baby, including spicy foods and vegetables in the cabbage family, as well as foods that might inhibit elimination in the mother.

This is definitely not an appropriate time to diet. Your body, especially if you are nursing, will naturally lose weight after birth. However, returning to your pre-pregnant size usually takes several months, at least. A healthy diet and moderate exercise over time will ensure this. Dieting only serves to deprive you and the baby of essential nutrients. If you have gained excessive weight during pregnancy, or simply want to be more trim than you are now, having just given birth, an excellent balanced diet is the best way to meet your goals. If weight or body image are of significant concern to you, speak with your midwife or doctor for information on how to eat right for breast feeding, or seek the assistance of a qualified nutritional consultant. Adjusting your diet to include healthful, high-quality foods protects your nutritional status, allows you to produce abundant milk, and helps get your weight under control. (See chapter 6 for specific ideas on diet and nutrition for lactating moms.)

❧ THE PARTNER RELATIONSHIP ☙

The days after birth can be confusing emotionally for your partner, and despite the incredible euphoria you both feel about the baby, this can be a challenging period in your relationship. During the pregnancy and birth, your partner may have had much anxiety about your well-being, along with his own set of performance concerns about the birth and his ability to support you emotionally and physically. Also, becoming a father adds an increased sense of responsibility to a man's life that can be at once welcomed and intimidating. Each successive baby is more responsibility. Emotional conflicts can arise as he integrates his own concerns and needs into your postpartum experience, particularly if you want him to drop everything to be with you and baby but he feels pressure to be at work, meeting his professional responsibilities. Internally, he too may wish to be home enjoying these exquisite hours with you but feels unable to do so.

Your partner may also feel overwhelmed and exhausted immediately after birth, especially if labor was long and arduous, or difficult. Add to this the sleep deprivation that your baby causes, and tensions may run high. Your own tumultuous emotions and increased physical needs place additional demand on him. Although this is natural, it may still be overwhelming for him. Let's hope he is sensitive and understanding of your physical and emotional needs, and can nurture you and enjoy this time with you. As much as you have energy to give him in return, he will appreciate your encouragement, praise, and love. A healthy marriage is a give-and-take of energy; he might need a bit of emotional support from you at this time as well. There is little attention paid to the demanding emotional changes that accompany becoming a father. Let him know you appreciate him—this will go a long way toward rejuvenating him emotionally as well.

❧ OLDER CHILDREN ☙

If you already have children, some of the challenges of the first days of postpartum won't be new to you. While each baby and thus each postpartum experience is different, it is likely that if this is your second baby—and certainly if this is your third child or more—certain things such as breast-feeding are remarkably easy for you. You've been through the steep learning curve of having a first child, and can rely more comfortably on the knowledge and skills you've already gained. However, you may be amazed at how gigantic and mature your older child now seems compared to your newborn!

With each new child come the joys and challenges of meeting the needs of your older children. Depending on the ages and temperaments of these kids, the transition may be more or less easy for you and for them.

Children over age 4 generally like to be active participants in newborn care; encourage help appropriate for their level, as this supports bonding among the children, and also allows the older ones to feel important and helpful. Give a lot of approval and keep criticism to a minimum. If you keep a watchful eye and stay nearby, even a toddler is unlikely to inflict more than a scratch to a newborn. Children over age 6 can be remarkably capable and helpful with a baby—even a newborn. Believe it or not, a lot of them even love to change diapers. One of my clients who recently gave birth has a 7-year-old daughter who wanted to be so involved and helpful that the mom finally had to say to her little girl, "This is *my* baby!" Nonetheless, this mom really appreciates how helpful her daughter is when she needs to grab a shower or start supper. The older child holds, plays with, changes, and loves the baby and Mom gets her work done.

If you have a toddler and are expecting a baby, your life is going to feel a bit out of control and overwhelming, particularly at first. This is why it's so important to have a strong network of friends and family—or hired help, if need be—to give you time to rest and focus on the baby, and to help your toddler receive the attention, interaction, and stimulation she often seems to need unless she is sleeping. It is also not uncommon for older kids, especially those in the 6 and under range, to suddenly start acting out. Remember to be understanding, even though you are tired and overwhelmed, and despite the fact that compared to a sweet little newborn, your older child suddenly seems tyrannical. Take a deep breath and let compassion wash over you. Having a little brother or sister can be as big a deal to your child as having a baby is to you. Enlist some help from Dad or another support person (who doesn't want to hold a newborn for an hour?) with the new baby if you have to, and spend a bit of quality time with your other child(ren). Just an hour here and there of focused attention without constant interruption from "you know who" can make your displaced child feel whole and important. This is also likely to encourage older children to welcome, rather than resent and reject, the baby.

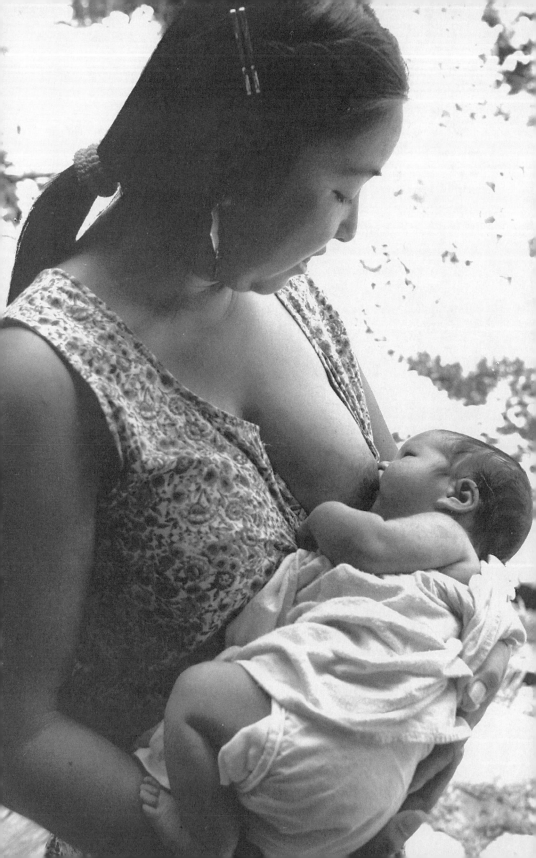

FIVE

The Next Six Weeks

*We need to recognize that there will inevitably be some stages and
seasons in our child's life that, at best, we'll just muddle through.*
Harriet Lerner, *The Mother Dance*

*I*t's astounding how many dramatic changes will occur in your body
and psyche in such a short time as the first 6 weeks after birth. According to an article in the medical journal *Women's Health,* "Recovery from childbirth is a complex process that may involve not only the gynecologic organs,
but also cardiovascular, respiratory, musculo-skeletal, urologic, gastrointestinal, endocrine, and nervous systems" (Gjerdingen et al., 1990). The changes
you undergo now are nothing short of an earthquake in your life. During the
first few days after birth, you're in a sort of suspended animation where time
takes on its own pace and meaning and a magical aura surrounds you and
the baby. Many new parents describe this period as surreal—it's hard to
believe the baby is really here and the birth, for which you have long prepared,
has already happened. Visitors come and go, your partner may be available full
time to help meet your needs and those of your other children, and the days
fly by as baby unfolds before your eyes, sleeping most of the time, waking up
for nourishment, then enjoying increasingly longer alert times.

After the first few days, some of the postbirth euphoria begins to fade
and reality sets in. As the Buddhist expression goes, "After enlightenment,
chop wood and carry water." By 10 days after the birth, your helpers will
probably have to go back to their own jobs and lives, the baby is starting to
be more expressive of his own needs, and older children may be wondering
"When is the baby going back to where he came from?" Although your
baby-bliss generally makes it all worthwhile, there may be moments of stress
when you wonder what were you thinking when you decided to have a baby.

According to Gjerdingen et al., "The process of postpartum recovery may span several months and is related to a variety of personal, family, and social variables" (1990). Viewing your needs during the postpartum as a continuum of your needs and baby's needs during pregnancy can remind you to take special care of yourself, and to allow others to care for you as well.

When you understand the normalcy of the changes you are experiencing, and employ some solid coping strategies, the second phase of your transition to motherhood during the first 6 weeks postpartum will be a lot smoother and saner.

❧ MORE BODY CHANGES ☙

By the second week after birth your bottom is starting to feel less tender, and if you have had a cesarean, some freedom of movement is beginning to return. In either case, you feel less sensitive and more mobile. You're probably beginning to get up and move around more, and you may have even seen your midwife or pediatrician for a follow-up visit. Your breasts have likely gotten quite full with milk, and if you are breast-feeding, your nipples may be tender.

You're definitely still physically aware that you've recently had a baby, but you have glimmers into what your body felt like before pregnancy and birth. However, looking in the mirror, your belly, hips, and derrière are still clear reminders of your voluptuous pregnant self. During pregnancy you may have felt good about gaining weight, and at the beginning of the second week postpartum you probably don't mind looking like you've just given birth, but by the end of the 6 weeks, perhaps you've had it. Many new mothers are beginning to wonder if they're ever going to have a waistline again, and the extra weight you still have may make you feel unattractive or without control of your body. This is a time for patience. Be grateful for your body's innate wisdom that knew to put on extra pounds to support you and baby through pregnancy and now into breast-feeding. Resume gentle exercise and remember that good food and moderate exercise will slowly but surely help you regain your shape.

Although you may feel terrific after giving birth, it is important to honor the major effort your body has just made. Take things slowly over these first 6 weeks. It is easy to overexert yourself, only to become drained and exhausted. This can happen quickly, such that even a small effort like fixing a meal requires you to lie down and rest. Throughout the first 6 weeks try not to lift anything much heavier than the baby and avoid lifting and pushing motions, such as hoisting groceries and running the vacuum. Such activities, if done too soon, can lead to increased postpartum bleeding to the point of hemorrhage during the first month after birth. In fact, the amount of bleeding you experience is an excellent indicator of the appropriate activity level for you. If your bleeding tapers off and then suddenly picks up after certain activities, this tells you to slow down—you're not yet ready for that level of exertion. During the first 6 weeks postpartum (at least!), push yourself to nap when the baby does, at least once daily. Becoming worn out can creep up on you—take care to prevent this from happening so you'll continue to feel well and relaxed during the early weeks after birth.

Recovery time is highly individual, and you may feel that by the end of 4 or 6 weeks you should be feeling more energetic for longer periods than you do. Yet you still tire easily, get suddenly and amazingly hungry, especially if you are breast-feeding, and may feel more aches and discomforts than you think you should. This is all natural, but many women are unprepared for the length of time it takes to return to "normal." Be patient, and give yourself plenty of time to adjust without judging your progress. You'll be able to enjoy your baby and your recuperation much more fully, and will ensure your health in the long run.

❧ WHERE DID EVERYBODY GO? . . . OR YES, ☙ YOU STILL NEED HELP AROUND THE HOUSE

During the pregnancy, emotional and tangible support provided by the spouse and others is related to the expectant mother's mental well-being...Mother's postpartum mental health is related to both the emotional and practical help (e.g., housework and child care activities) provided by the husbands and others.

Gjerdingen 1991

After a couple of weeks, your mom or sister has to go back to her own home and responsibilities, friends have their own households to care for, your husband must return to work, and the time for which you hired the doula has expired. So now you are 2 weeks postpartum and home alone with the baby, probably feeling not quite ready to be back into the swing of caring fully for both of you. If you have prepared wisely, you have staggered your postpartum care so you have full-time help from family and friends for the first couple of weeks, with part-time help available for a few weeks after. This is particularly important if this is not your first baby, and there are toddlers or elementary school-aged children to care for.

At 2 weeks postpartum you can expect to feel well enough to be on your feet for an hour or so at a stretch, long enough to heat leftovers or prepare a simple meal, give a toddler a bath, wash a few dishes, or toss a load of laundry into the washer. But you should not do all of these things in one morning or evening by yourself. You still need help. Therefore, it is important to plan ahead, determining in advance who can come in and help you with some of your responsibilities, perhaps giving your toddler a bath, or cleaning up dinner while you give the bath. It would be great if friends and family continued to bring meals occasionally into the first months postpartum, or at least you can help your husband devise menus that are simple to prepare, nutritious, and yield abundant, easy-to-reheat, tasty leftovers.

Be gentle on yourself when you find you need help doing things you thought you'd be ready to do by now, and which just a year ago you did easily. Your body has put out a tremendous amount of energy, you are operating on significant sleep deprivation, and if you are breast-feeding, you are expending an enormous amount of caloric energy to feed the baby. It is natural to tire easily, and to continue to need more rest for several months to come. It is common for mothers even several months after the birth to fall asleep at 8 P.M., nursing the baby or getting a toddler down for a night's sleep. I myself have mumbled through many a bedtime story, even well into the first year after a birth.

❧ REINVENTING YOURSELF ❧ AS A MOTHER

When you give birth, you do so not only to a baby and to a family, but also to a new facet of yourself. For most women, the first week or two after birth goes by in a sort of mystical haze, but as the reality of lost sleep, leaking breasts, and too-tight clothes sets in, you may find yourself wondering just who and where you are in all of it. Sometime toward the end of that first month or 6 weeks postpartum, you may find yourself wondering what you were thinking by having a baby—or yet another baby, if you already have one or more children. And the amazing beauty of motherhood is that you can experience many feelings at once—pure and all encompassing love for your baby and complete emotional crisis about being a mother. Sally Placksin describes postpartum as an "endless blur of day and night" with diapers, dishes, sleepless nights, and leaking breasts flowing into one another. You may feel you were made for more than this. If you are accustomed to being in control and well put together, leaky boobs and an inconsolably crying baby can feel overwhelming. One mother I worked with many years ago, formerly a psychiatric nurse as well as a skilled artist and business manager, confided that she felt utterly incompetent caring for a newborn though she'd previously managed the care of many patients at a large hospital along with her husband's successful business.

As your visitors return to their daily lives, you may feel a sense of loss and grieving over the attention you received while you were pregnant and that helped shape your identity and expectations as a mother. Your life has dramatically and permanently changed, and you want everyone else's perception of you to support this shift. If this doesn't happen you might feel overlooked and unrecognized. You want the whole world to beam with you, to share this incredible transformation you're going through, but after a couple of weeks the whole world has gone back to its mundane reality, sometimes leaving a new mother feeling isolated in her experience.

Allowing yourself to experience this multitude of feelings is much healthier than trying to deny them. In fact, stuffing them up inside because you feel ashamed or guilty and have conflicting feelings about motherhood can be damaging to your health and may lead to a crisis of postpartum depression. Instead, find ways to express your conflicts, whether by keeping a journal, talking to a friend, or talking to an understanding healthcare provider (preferably one who is a mother herself), or find other creative or artistic outlets. All these can be a relief and help you to discover your identity and voice in the chaos of new motherhood.

Becoming a mother puts women face to face with their ideals and judgments, just when they are feeling vulnerable and overwhelmed. Some women develop greater compassion for their own mother; others feel terrified they will repeat what they perceive as mistakes their mother made. A new mother also tends to compare herself to other mothers, believing that others are more competent or capable, as she feels completely overwhelmed. You may also feel bumbling. It's unfortunate that too often the difficulties of new motherhood are glossed over. It can be an awesome responsibility to take care of a newborn, especially if you expected it was going to be a honeymoon after birth. It can take weeks, even months, to get comfortable and confident with your baby and your role as mother.

New motherhood puts you on a steep learning curve—so steep that you may feel inadequate to the climb, or that for every step forward you slide back two. But eventually you get comfortable with the terrain, and you reach new vistas and plateaus. Talking with others who are honest about their experience as new parents can help you recognize that you are not the first to climb this mountain, and that with the proper tools and patience, you will survive.

❧ MORE BIRTH REFLECTIONS ☙

Now that you're gaining a little distance from your birth, you may have new insights or feelings—some of which are incredibly joyous and others of which include disappointment, anger, or resentment. If you haven't already written your birth story, this is an excellent time to create an account of the experience. Even if all the details weren't your ideal, this story will be an important piece of history for your child, as well as a good way for you to process your own feelings about the experience. If you continue to have lingering feelings of sadness or disappointment about your birth, speak with a supportive and understanding friend, counselor, or care provider about what happened. Releasing pent-up emotions is much healthier than carrying them around as a permanent part of your personal fabric.

Birth experiences can form the basis for meaningful creative projects, whether a book of thoughts or reflections on birth, a painting, a dance. Even if you can't physically create something because of your schedule with a newborn, envision what you would do to honor and celebrate the experience of your birth.

❧ FURTHER BREAST-FEEDING ADVENTURES ☙

Breast feeding is a profoundly intimate and potentially very satisfying experience that is shared between a mother and baby. Indeed, it is an undeniably sensual experience that can be highly pleasurable for the nursing "couple." Unfortunately, we live in a culture that has skewed sexual values and perceptions of women's bodies. We at once allow billboards, newsstands, movies, television, and CD covers to show images of barely clad women in sexually suggestive postures and settings, while ostracizing, harassing, and expelling from public institutions women who dare to breast-feed in public. Sally Placksin writes: "Many factors currently exist that threaten to sabotage breastfeeding moms." Among these are the public opinion that it is an inappropriate relationship for the mother and baby to maintain past a certain time (perhaps the first few months). The disdain for the existence of something that could be construed as a sexual experience between mother and baby is evident when a breast-feeding mother is told at a family gathering that "perhaps she'd be more comfortable nursing in the bedroom." Even at the public zoo, the breast-feeding area is near the public rest rooms. The message is that it's okay to see women's breasts objectified as sexual objects in the media; we just can't see the breasts of nursing mothers.

Hospital routines and attitudes may also present a significant obstacle to the breast-feeding mother from the start, as discussed earlier, undermining her confidence in her ability to feed her baby. One of my home-birth clients recently remarked that now that she was nursing her baby, she saw the sample formula pack that hospitals provide as a hidden message of "planned failure" for breast feeding. "Here," she said, emulating the attitude, "take this just in case you really can't do it." This attitude can haunt you over the first few weeks, as you wonder, in spite of the fact that your baby is growing before your eyes, whether the baby is getting adequate nourishment from your breast. There has actually been an international effort to counteract negative hospital attitudes and practices that can interfere with breast-feeding success. Known as the Baby-Friendly Hospital Initiative, it is an effort to promote hospital environments that support mothers in their desire to breast-feed. An international standard was published jointly in 1989 by the World Health Organization (WHO) and the United Nations Children's Fund (UNICEF). This statement, entitled *Protecting, Promoting, and Supporting Breast-feeding: The Special Role of Maternity Services,* had the support of other international organizations as well. Baby-friendly hospitals are those that implement all of the Ten Steps to Successful Breastfeeding, and receive certificates of recognition. Ask your hospital or care provider if she is familiar with or part of the Baby-Friendly Hospital Initiative when you make your care-provider choices during pregnancy.

TEN STEPS TO SUCCESSFUL BREAST FEEDING

Every facility providing maternity services and care for newborn infants should:

1. Have a written breast-feeding policy that is routinely communicated to all health care staff.

2. Train all health care staff in skills necessary to implement this policy.

3. Inform all pregnant women about the benefits of breast-feeding within a half-hour of birth.

4. Help mothers initiate breast feeding within a half-hour of birth.

5. Show mothers how to breast-feed, and how to maintain lactation even if they should be separated from their infants.

6. Give newborn infants no food or drink other than breast milk unless *medically* indicated.

7. Practice rooming-in—allow mothers and infants to remain together 24 hours a day.

8. Encourage breast-feeding on demand.

9. Give no artificial teats or pacifiers to breast-feeding infants.

10. Foster the establishment of breast-feeding support groups and refer mothers to them on discharge from the hospital or clinic.

DID YOU KNOW . . .

The International Code of Marketing of Breastmilk Substitutes prohibits:

- Free samples to mothers
- Advertising to the public
- Promotion in healthcare facilities
- Gifts or samples to health workers
- Words and pictures that idealize bottle feeding
- Advice to mothers by company sales staff

Countries that have adopted this code, along with other measures to promote, protect, and support breast feeding, have seen a doubling of breast-feeding rates in urban areas.

Do your care providers know about this code?

From *Protecting, Promoting, and Supporting Breast-feeding: The Special Role of Maternity Services*, WHO/UNICEF, Geneva, Switzerland, 1989

Husbands must also understand and serve as your primary support and protector as you build your breast-feeding relationship with your baby. The widespread practice of bottle feeding has established an expectation that everyone should be able to have a hand in feeding the baby, and that breast feeding somehow deprives fathers of an essential ability to nurture the baby. Furthermore, fathers may become extremely anxious and upset over a crying baby, being all too ready to substitute a bottle for the breast to pacify the baby. Their own mother, and your mother, if they are not veteran breast-feeders themselves, may add to the pressure, encouraging your husband to bring you to your senses and give the baby a bottle. After all, they may say, you were both bottle-fed and you turned out just fine. Fathers need to understand the benefits of breast feeding and the subtle but clear role their support or lack of it plays in your ability to nurse successfully and for a prolonged time. They must learn to accept your primary role of feeding the baby while establishing their own ways of being close to their newborn. They must also learn to embrace the earthiness of your body functions, which may include some milk let-down when you are physically intimate with each other. (See page 107 for further discussion of this matter.)

Although breast feeding is probably getting easier for you now in the first weeks after birth, it still requires perseverance. Breast-feeding success depends on the mother feeling confident about her ability to nourish her baby. It is therefore still important to have someone you can talk with about breast feeding if you become anxious or concerned, or if you hit any trouble spots. Books about breast feeding provide some support, but a mother who has breast-fed successfully is an indispensable ally. If you don't know any women who have breast-fed successfully whom you feel you can call, contact La Leche League (1-800-LA-LECHE) for a directory of breast-feeding support groups in your area. Meeting other breast-feeding mothers will give you enough support to make your own experience satisfying and rewarding.

℀ CARING FOR YOUR BREASTS ℀

Some of the most common breast-feeding problems in the first few weeks are sore nipples, engorgement, and actual concerns about the baby's feeding habits, all of which have been addressed in previous chapters. As this point, your breasts are probably quite full of milk, and are apt to be heavy and leaking often. A good bra that provides adequate support and easy access for nursing is an indispensable aid. Most department stores now carry maternity bras, and there are also a number of mail-order catalogs specializing in clothing for nursing mothers (see Resources). Make sure your bra fits well, as a constricting bra can lead to plugged milk ducts and mastitis (see below) and inadequate support doesn't do much of anything for you. Cotton is the best fabric for nursing bras, as it is both absorbent and breathes well, reducing the incidence of thrush on the nipples.

Similarly, if you choose to use nursing pads inside your bra to absorb leaking milk, do so only when necessary, such as when you are at work or a special function, and wear only cotton nursing pads. Change and wash your bras every day or two, and dry them in the dryer or in the sun occasionally to kill any yeast that might thrive in them, particularly if you have had a problem with thrush.

MASTITIS

Milk flows through ducts—little channels in your breasts—before it exits through the nipples. These channels may become blocked when a breast is engorged with milk or from physical constriction, which can occur from sleeping on the breast when it is full or from wearing a too-snug bra. Blocked ducts are also more common when women have been overdoing it—that is, running around too much without attention to adequate rest, fluids, and nutrition.

Plugged ducts can become inflamed quickly and unexpectedly, causing severe discomfort. Some localized discomfort, a hard red knot, and a streaky red area on your breast where the discomfort is centered are the first symptoms you're likely to notice. Fever, chills, malaise, dizziness, nausea, and general flulike symptoms then quickly follow. This condition is commonly referred to as *mastitis,* or breast infection. It is preventable, and if caught and treated early, it will usually clear up within 24 hours. Untreated, it can lead to a breast abscess with a more serious systemic infection. Don't let it go that far!

Mothers who are very active or overtired are especially likely to develop mastitis. Perhaps this is because they aren't settling down long enough to nurse the baby until the breasts are emptied or because fatigue lowers overall immunity. Plugged ducts are even more apt to occur when moms are not consuming enough fluids and eating healthy meals. If you've been overdoing it, slow down! If you notice any of the signs of breast inflammation, stop everything! Put on loose, warm, comfortable clothing; jump into bed or relax in a cozy chair with your baby and a cup of hot tea or broth; and observe all treatment recommendations that apply to you.

Discuss any fever or infection that occurs within the first weeks after birth with your healthcare provider. Fever accompanied by abdominal tenderness or foul-smelling vaginal discharge could be a uterine infection ("childbed fever"), which is very dangerous for the mother. Seek help immediately.

TO TREAT MASTITIS NATURALLY

Rest, fluids, and nourishment, along with frequent nursing of the baby on the affected side, are the primary treatments for a plugged duct and the best prevention and cure of mastitis. With the following suggestions you should notice improvement in 6 to 12 hours and complete recovery within 24 hours. You may notice slight discomfort (a sore or bruised feeling) for up to several days longer. If you do, continue the internal remedies until you are completely well.

- Drink a tall glass of water (warm or at room temperature) every waking hour of the day. This is incredibly important! Sip on catnip tea to ease stress, tension, and discomfort.

- Eat very well, especially hearty grain and vegetable soups. Miso paste, made from soybeans, is particularly nourishing and is a beneficial addition to an unsalted soup stock. Add 3 tablespoons of miso paste per quart of stock, or to taste.

- Take naps throughout the day. Have no visitors or social activities until you are completely recovered. If you relapse into fatigue, the problem can easily recur.

- Nurse your baby often on the affected side in order to drain the ducts thoroughly and to flush the breast. It may feel uncomfortable to suckle the baby on the painful breast, but doing so will shorten the duration of the blockage. Nursing the baby on the side with the infection is perfectly safe. However, if an abscess occurs anywhere near the nipple, nurse on the other breast and hand-express from the affected side.

- Use compresses and tub soaks to apply moist heat to your breasts. Fill a sink or basin with hot water and hang your breast into it as you gently massage the blockage toward the nipple. Use gingerroot, chamomile, marsh mallow root, burdock root, and slippery elm infusions as compresses. Hot water will suffice if nothing else is available.

- Apply a poultice of freshly grated raw potato (just a regular baker or boiler will do) 2 or 3 times a day. This is a wonderful remedy because nearly everyone has a potato, and it is remarkably effective in reducing pain, blockage, and inflammation. Remove the poultice when it becomes warm, usually after about 20 minutes.

- Take $1/2$ to 1 teaspoon of echinacea tincture every 2 to 4 hours, depending on the severity of the problem. Continue for at least 24 hours after all signs of illness are past. This is perfectly safe for baby.

> ⤙ Take 500 mg of vitamin C every 2 to 4 hours. You may notice that your baby's poops become looser, but this is of no concern.
>
> ⤙ If you have a fever, drink hot elder blossom and spearmint infusion ($^1/_2$ ounce of each herb steeped for 20 minutes in a quart of boiling water). Keep drinking it until you break a sweat, up to 2 quarts. Stay warm under the covers.
>
> ⤙ In the rare event that an abscess develops, seek professional help. Many abscesses can be treated at home, but in serious cases you should consult an experienced health care practitioner.

❧ HERBS AND BREAST FEEDING ❧

When you are breast-feeding, much of what you take into your body you give to your baby along with your milk. This includes many pharmaceutical drugs, both prescription and over the counter (OTC), as well as many herbs. And just because herbs are natural, that doesn't mean they're all safe for you or the baby. As with pharmaceutical substances, some medicines might be fine for adults but not so for babies and children. Therefore, it is important to know that what you ingest while nursing is safe for both of you.

There are many resources for learning about what medications are safe to take or must be avoided when you are breast-feeding (see *The Breastfeeding Book*, by William and Martha Sears), but it can be harder to determine which herbs are considered safe while nursing. According to *The Botanical Safety Handbook* (McGuffin et al. 1997), nationally recognized as the definitive guide to herb safety, herbs are classified as follows:

Class 1: Herbs that can be safely consumed when used appropriately

Class 2: Herbs for which special restrictions apply, unless otherwise directed by an expert qualified in the use of the described substance

2a: For external use only

2b: Not to be used during pregnancy

2c: Not to be used while nursing

2d: Other specific use restrictions as noted

Class 3: Herbs for which significant data exist to recommend labeling "To be used only under the supervision of an expert qualified in the use of this substance"

Class 4: Herbs for which insufficient data are available for classification

The herbs recommended in this book generally fall into Class 1, unless otherwise noted. Class 2c herbs, those "not to be used *(internally)* while nursing unless otherwise directed by an expert qualified in the appropriate use of this substance," are as follows:

Alkanet	Comfrey
Aloe vera	Elecampane
Aloes	Ephedra
Basil*	Garlic*
Black cohosh	Joe Pye
Bladderwrack	Licorice**
Borage	Male fern
Bugleweed	Purging buckthorn
Cascara sagrada	Senna
Chinese rhubarb	Stillingia
Coltsfoot	Wormwood

In addition to the herbs on this list, breast-feeding mothers should avoid all herbs with known toxicity, herbs that have active hormonal properties, herbs that are stimulants or strong sedatives, and the internal use of essential oils. Dr. Tieraona Low Dog, a family physician, herbalist, and midwife, recommends avoiding the following herbs in addition to the above list: cinchona bark, cola seeds, guarana, jasmine flowers, kava kava, madder root, pulsatilla, and senecio.

NOURISHING HERBS FOR THE POSTPARTUM MOTHER

A number of herbs that are excellent for supporting your physical and emotional well-being can also be safely taken by the breast-feeding mother. Indeed, several such herbs actually help to support breast-milk production and quality. Herbs that are nourishing are sometimes known as *nutritive* herbs; those that support the nervous system, helping to relieve stress and tension, are called *nervines;* and those that promote breast milk are referred to as *galactagogues.* Nutritive herbs can also be tonics. One of the beauties of herbs is that one plant can have many actions and serve many functions.

---

* May be used as a culinary seasoning *(author's note)*

** May be used as directed in this book in specific formulas *(author's note)*

Nutritive (Tonic) Herbs

- **Alfalfa.** Alfalfa is a good source of chlorophyll and a nutrient-rich herb. Liquid chlorophyll, derived from alfalfa, is an excellent blood tonic, enhancing iron levels and reducing postpartum anemia.

- **Ashwaganda.** An herb from the tradition of Indian Ayurvedic medicine, ashwaganda enjoys wide acceptance in the herbal community in the United States to help us adapt to stress; thus, it is classified as an herbal *adaptogen*. These herbs gently support the adrenal system, reducing irritability and jangled nerves, while serving as a gentle support to the immune system. It is generally taken as a tincture or as a tea with a small amount of milk and honey.

  Dose: $^1/_2$–1 teaspoon tincture 2 times daily; tea 1–2 cups daily

- **Gotu kola.** This is another herb that hails from the Ayurvedic medical tradition of India. It is known as both a tonic for the connective tissue, making it excellent to include in formulas for restoring uterine ligament tone, and a nervous system and cerebral tonic par excellence. As such, it is said to reduce nervous exhaustion and promote mental clarity. Use it in teas or take as an herbal tincture.

  Combine with ashwaganda as well as any of the nervines described below, to benefit the nervous system.

  Dose: As for ashwaganda

- **Hawthorn berries, leaves, and flowers.** Typically, hawthorn is used as a tonic herb for the heart, and indeed it provides many benefits to the cardiac system. I frequently blend the berries, leaves, and flowers in formulas for stress reduction and overall gentle tonification. They combine well in teas and tinctures with lemon balm, rose hips, hibiscus, and spearmint, making a flavorful and refreshing beverage and medicine.

  Dose: 1 teaspoon tincture twice daily or 1–2 cups tea daily

- **Milky oats.** These make a nourishing tonic for the nervous system. Oats themselves have long been used as a healthful food for mothers and children, being very high in vitamins and minerals. Oats are also known to provide vigor and energy to horses. In the form of the tincture of the fresh, milky seeds of the plant, a new mother can take oats over a long period, even many months, to provide gentle calm.

  Dose: Take as tincture, $^1/_2$–1 teaspoon, 1–3 times daily

- **Nettle.** This herb is particularly nutritive, containing trace minerals and vitamins, especially iron, potassium, and silica. It is used to treat anemia and weakness and to stabilize blood sugar. It is especially called for if you are feeling stressed or physically or emotionally drained (or both). Nettle tea is delicious alone or in combination with other herbs such as alfalfa, rose, and spearmint. Nettle is also used as an antihistaminic herb, reducing allergic reactions when there is a tendency toward chronic allergies, especially hay fever.

  Dose: Take 1–3 cups daily. Prepare by steeping $1/2$ ounce dried herb per 2 cups boiling water for 30 minutes.

- **Red raspberry leaf.** Known mostly as a prenatal tonic, this is actually a general nutritive herb that makes an excellent beverage tea. It is rich in minerals, tonifying to the uterus, and a pleasant addition to teas. Combines well with nettles, mint, rose hips, and many other beverage herbs.

  Dose: Dosage and preparation same as for nettle

- **Rose hips.** Both fresh and dried, rose hips provide a flavorful and plentiful source of vitamin C. They imbue a rich red color to tea, and impart a delightful tart flavor. Delicious with hibiscus, nettle, raspberry, hawthorn, lemon balm, and spearmint.

  Dose: Add 1 teaspoon–1 tablespoon herb to other teas for flavor

Nervines

- **Ashwagandha.** See page 144.

- **Catnip.** Catnip enjoys a strong reputation for use for mothers and by mothers for their children. Its gentle but reliable relaxing qualities make it an appropriate nervine for new mothers, and these qualities, much as with chamomile, lavender, and other aromatic herbs, are imparted to the baby, helping reduce colic and fussiness. Its mild taste enhances a tea, but it is also effective in tincture form.

  Dose: 1–4 cups of tea or $1/2$–1 teaspoon tincture 3–4 times daily. Prepare by steeping 1 tablespoon dried herb in 1 cup boiling water for 10 minutes.

- **Chamomile.** This herb relaxes the mother, and, through the breast milk, provides gentle relaxation to the baby. Taken by the mother, it can also help to allay milk colic symptoms in the baby. Although you can take chamomile as a tincture, it is best to drink as a tea, steeped for only 10 minutes to ensure a pleasant flavor. It is frequently combined with other gentle nervines such as catnip and lavender. Take daily, either throughout the day or shortly before bed to promote a restful sleep.

Dose: Dosage and preparation same as for catnip

- **Hops.** We know hops as a primary ingredient in beermaking, but it is also a strong relaxing herb. It is reserved for use when there is insomnia, and should not be used when there is depression. It can help when there is difficulty relaxing enough to allow an effective milk let-down reflex. Generally taken as a tincture, it is also a mild bitter digestive tonic for gas and bloating and irritable bowels.

    Dose: $1/2$ teaspoon tincture 1–3 times daily

- **Lavender.** This lovely herb lends itself well to teas and can be used in tinctures, both forms providing deep but gentle relaxing actions for the nervous system. It is beneficial when there is difficulty sleeping, and is often combined with chamomile, fennel seed, and catnip to enhance breast-milk production and the let-down reflex. Sipping the tea imparts the aromatherapy benefits of inhaled lavender oil, and is a sensory treat.

    Dose: Prepare tea as for catnip and chamomile. Tincture dosage same as for hops.

- **Lemon balm.** Classically known as the "gladdening herb" because of its uplifting effects on the mood and emotions, it is a gentle nervous system tonic, typically used as a beverage tea. Its delicate lemony flavor blends well with other herbal teas, and when used by breastfeeding mothers, its calming effects are conveyed to the baby through the breast milk.

    Dose: Preparation and dosage same as for chamomile and catnip

- **Milky oats.** See above.

- **Motherwort.** This bitter but effective herb helps to reduce tension levels in new mothers. In fact, the name *motherwort* implies that it is a healing herb for mothers (*wort* means "herbaceous plant"). The botanical name, *Leonurus cardiaca,* means "lion-hearted" and reflects its use for strengthening the cardiovascular system. In particular, it is excellent for reducing nervous heart palpitations and anxiety, and for taking the edge off jangled nerves and irritability. Furthermore, motherwort is a uterine tonic, and can be used to help the uterus return to its nonpregnant size and allay the pain associated with postpartum uterine cramps. Because of its bitter taste, it is best to take as a tincture. Combine with other nervine herbs or take singly.

Dose: 1/2 teaspoon 2–4 times daily

❧ **Skullcap.** Use skullcap short or long term to support the nervous system, reduce tension, promote restful sleep, and treat irritability and mild forms of postnatal blues, the result of inadequate sleep, exhaustion, and overstimulation. Generally taken as a tincture, it combines well with many other nervines and tonics.

Dose: 1/2–1 teaspoon 2–4 times daily

❧ **Vervain.** This herb helps the mother who is at once irritable and weepy (ever yelled at your husband or child or slammed a door and then burst out crying?). It is generally combined with other herbs such as milky oats and skullcap in tincture form, and it can be taken for several months at a time. It is excellent for treating the emotional symptoms of premenstrual syndrome.

Dose: 1/2–1 teaspoon 2–3 times daily

Galactagogues

❧ **Blessed thistle.** This herb has a long history in promoting breast milk in new mothers. It also has properties that help allay uterine bleeding, making it an all-around generally beneficial herb for the postpartum mother in the first few weeks. It can help offset mild irritability, and is also a good general digestive tonic, particularly when there is sluggish digestion. As it is bitter, take as a tincture.

Dose: 1/2 teaspoon 3 times daily

❧ **Dandelion leaf.** Much like nettle, this is a highly nutritive green plant, being rich in trace minerals and iron. The best way to take dandelion leaf to promote breast milk is as a fresh green vegetable cooked with a bit of lemon and butter for flavor, taken several times per week. The fresh spring greens are the least bitter and make delicious eating. Use in tincture form for treating constipation.

Dose: Take 1 teaspoon twice daily

❧ **Fennel.** Another herb classically listed among those that promote breast milk, fennel has a mild, pleasant taste. It makes a palatable tea, or use as a pleasant flavoring for other, more bitter tinctures for promoting milk. (See also vervain and vitex.) Steep 1 tsp. seeds in 1 cup boiling water for 10 minutes.

Dose: 1–2 cups tea daily

- **Fenugreek.** This herb has long been used to encourage milk production. Take as a warm tea while trying to establish or improve the milk supply. You may take it alone or in combination with other galactagogues and nervines, and it may also be used in tincture form. Prepare same as for fennel.

- **Nettle.** This is perhaps my favorite herb to use for enriching and enhancing breast-milk production, while providing optimal nutrients and energy for the mother. I often recommend it in large quantities— as much as 1 quart of strong tea daily—as an adjunct part of the diet, but even a cup or two daily, several times a week, will bring significant benefit to the overall well-being of the mother. Nettle can also be eaten as a fresh green, but be careful of the sting during preparation. Cooking destroys the sting.

- **Saw palmetto.** Though primarily touted as an herb for the treatment of male reproductive system troubles, saw palmetto also earns praise for its use as a reproductive tonic for women, enhancing libido, relieving fatigue, and promoting increased milk flow. It should be used short term by nursing mothers, generally for not longer than 6 weeks at a time, and is generally prescribed in tincture or capsule form. It combines well with many of the other nutritive tonics and galactagogues described in this section.

  Dose: $1/2$ teaspoon tincture twice daily

- **Vervain.** In addition to being a nervine, vervain is listed in many herbal texts as one that promotes lactation. As it is bitter, it is best to use in tincture form. It combines well with vitex, ashwaganda, and licorice root in tincture form.

- **Vitex.** The use for the promotion of breast milk is a controversial topic. Traditionally, midwives and herbalists have used it for this purpose for many centuries. However, modern research indicates that vitex actually inhibits prolactin, the hormone that promotes breast-milk production. Nonetheless, many midwives and herbalists still consider it a valuable adjunct in establishing breast feeding when there is difficulty with breast-milk production. Certainly, further clinical research must be done to determine the helpfulness of its use in this capacity. Modern naturopathic physician and midwife Mary Bove of Brattleboro, Vermont, has suggested in personal communications that the research done on prolactin inhibition was not done on lactating women, and thus the physiology of what occurs when prolactin is naturally elevated, as with breastfeeding, may be vastly different. She feels this may account for the discrepancy between traditional use for lactating populations and scientific studies in nonlactating women. Vitex can often be used with benefit when there are postnatal blues that are hormonally related. It is almost always used in tincture form, though capsules are also available.

Dose: 1 teaspoon tincture twice daily

 Energy Pick-Me-Up

Nutritive and tonifying to the nervous system, this tea provides energy without being a stimulant. It provides trace minerals and can be safely taken when you need a little energy boost, or better yet, taken regularly as an excellent dietary supplement and tonic.

$^1/_2$ ounce dried nettle leaf

$^1/_2$ ounce red raspberry leaf

$^1/_4$ ounce gotu kola leaf

$^1/_4$ ounce spearmint leaf or rosemary leaf (your choice)

To prepare, steep 1 tablespoon per cup of boiling water for 20 minutes, then strain.

Dose: Take as a tea, 1–2 cups daily

CHINESE TONIC HERBS FOR POSTPARTUM

During the weeks and months postpartum, you may find that sleep deprivation, stress, and the energy requirements of parenting a newborn, especially if you are breast-feeding, leave you feeling somewhat drained. Deep-acting herbal medicines can help revitalize and protect your system from stress and depletion. The following Chinese herbal remedy is good for nurturing the blood and revitalizing the core energy of the body, and may be taken as a postpartum tonic. Used when you have a pallid or sallow complexion and suffer from reduced appetite, fatigue, lightheadedness, and possibly palpitations and anxiety. It is available in prepared form (see Resources), which is more palatable to most Americans than is the tea, or make it into a decoction as directed.

Eight-Treasure Formula

   3 grams actractylodes
   3 grams dang gui
   3 grams ginseng
   3 grams ligusticum
   3 grams peony
   3 grams poria
   3 grams rehmannia
   $1\frac{1}{2}$ grams honey-fried licorice

Simmer all of the herbs in 4 cups of water for 1 hour. Strain the liquid from the herbs and store in a glass jar. Return the herbs to the cooking pot and add 2 cups of water. Simmer for 30 minutes and strain, adding this liquid to the first batch of liquid. Cool to room temperature and store in the refrigerator. Will keep refrigerated for 3 days.

Dose: Drink 1 cup of the tea, 2 times daily, or the prepared product as directed.

Note: Although these herbs are not stimulants, they are very warming to the system. Thus, they are too stimulating for some babies who by nature are already very warm. Should your baby become irritable or develop a rash while you are taking these herbs, discontinue immediately. The rash will clear when you stop taking the herbs.

THE MAGIC OF YOUR BABY

Even now, weeks after your baby has been born, you may find yourself amazed at how connected you still feel to her. The movements your baby makes may remind you of the movements she made while in your belly, as indeed they are similar. Your baby's scents and sounds have become imprinted on your soul, and within a matter of seconds you can marvel not only at the newness of your baby but also at the feeling that this child has always been with you, always been a part of you. As you are aware of your intense feelings of connection to this child, you may also experience feelings of vulnerability for the baby. It is no cliché that mothers wear their hearts outside of their bodies. Your passionate attachment may at times bring you to tears in the early weeks after birth, as no doubt it will many times over the course of your life.

You may also feel an increased sense of vulnerability about older children as they go out into the world unprotected by the constant presence of your arms as this baby is now protected. Indeed, many new mothers express that they suddenly found themselves anxious or had paranoid thoughts about an older child when he ventured from home. Perhaps maternal awareness is so heightened during this time that we feel unusually open and vulnerable. This is all part of the beautiful and terrifying territory of maternal love.

During the first weeks, you are both instinctively and intentionally developing familiarity with your baby's signals, trying to understand the meaning of different cries, gestures, and facial expressions. At times you'll be gratified by your quick and easy ability to satisfy and comfort your baby; at other times you'll feel overwhelmed and frustrated by your seeming inability to console or pacify your crying baby. You're also probably trying to get a sense of the baby's rhythms and patterns, but at this point they probably change as quickly as you recognize them. During this time babies begin to wake from a sort of post-birth dream world and start to show more of their neediness—this happens, of course, just when all of your help goes back to work.

The blissful times will take care of themselves, but for the stressful times, it is important to develop coping skills so that you don't become exhausted and exasperated. It's a really terrible thing, but it is only when women become mothers and experience the intensity of exhaustion, frustration, and rage—the emotional counterpoints of supreme maternal bliss—that they recognize that the potential for child abuse exists within every individual who is pushed too far with too few reserves or opportunities for support and help. It is not uncommon for a new mother, exhausted and frustrated, to say to her husband, "You'd better come take this baby before I do something rash." While generally said in jest, such feelings of helplessness can be powerful and overwhelming. Adrienne Rich, in her classic book *Of Woman Born*, provides an eloquent, honest, and moving presentation of the varied emotions mothers go through. I highly recommend this book to women who are learning to cope with the tremendous range of feelings they have as they become mothers. Honoring our feelings while developing coping skills for dealing with a fussy baby is the most constructive approach to dealing with the difficulties of motherhood.

TIPS FOR COPING WITH CONFLICTING EMOTIONS

- ✌ Remember, almost all mothers feel conflicting emotions about motherhood, whether or not they admit it.
- ✌ Conflicting feelings are a natural response to the stresses of a job, which no matter how rewarding, is also demanding.

❧ Conflicting feelings don't mean you're a bad mother or that you don't love your baby.

❧ Find outlets for your stress, confusion, or frustration. Keep a journal, talk to a trusted friend or family member, take a walk, speak with your midwife or other care provider, get involved in a creative endeavor such as an art class, get a massage, or go to the bookstore for an hour.

❧ Remember that babies are not deliberately demanding; they just have limited ways of expressing their needs. If your baby is fussing and there is nothing hurting her, her diaper is dry, and she is well fed, provide comfort and see if that helps. If it doesn't, you have done your best. Simply put the baby down in a safe place or hand her over to your husband, and take 15 minutes away from the sound of her crying. Get something to eat, take a shower, make yourself some tea. By now someone else may have had some luck, but if not, you'll approach the baby with fresh energy and enthusiasm.

The impulse to lose patience with a baby is not uncommon. You may be more tired than you realize, you may feel trapped and isolated, and your blood sugar or hormones are fluctuating greatly. If you are losing your patience, put the baby down in her crib, go outside, and try to relax. If you can't, call a friend to come over. If this is happening on a regular basis and you're genuinely concerned you might hurt your baby, talk to someone you trust and please seek professional help. You might simply have postpartum depression, which is treatable and nothing to be ashamed about.

❧ FUSSY BABIES ❧

Babies get fussy and cry just because they are babies and that's how they express themselves. Perhaps your baby was startled by a sudden noise or movement; has a wet or soiled diaper; is hungry, cold, or overheated; or just needs touching, holding, or comfort. A baby's screaming can be quite dramatic, especially to you as the mother, because your hormones are intricately responsive to the baby's needs.

Part of becoming a mother is learning the fine art of dispassion. This is the ability to step back and evaluate what is going on with your child. It is a particularly useful skill to develop and will come in handy when your child is 6 and whining and crying over that toy she really wants in the grocery store or the cute kitten she wants to adopt. In a sense, you learn when to take the crying seriously and when to let it roll over you even as you provide a steady source of support and comfort. It requires the art of knowing your child's cues and having confidence in your own judgment.

If you've determined that your baby's basic needs are met, and that he's just expressing discontent, one of the best things to do is bundle him up, put him in a baby sling, and go for a walk (Daddy can take baby for a walk if you're not up for it). You can do this in virtually any weather short of a thunderstorm, as long as the baby is bundled up if it is cold. Walking and rocking motions are soothing for babies, and most babies calm down when taken outdoors.

Colic is another common reason for fussiness. Colic is a catchall term for a condition in which a baby is fussy, uncomfortable, or downright distressed, despite being dry, warm, well fed, and comforted. It may be caused by gas in the baby's intestines, or it may just be part of getting used to digestion and other bodily functions. Colic is a difficult experience not only for the baby but also for the parents, who find it worrisome and exhausting to have an inconsolable baby. Some babies seem more prone to colic than others. It generally begins around 2 weeks after birth, and most outgrow it by 4 months.

Sometimes colic is going to happen no matter what you do because your baby's digestive tract is just learning to work smoothly. Do your best to prevent it, and comfort your baby if it arises. Create calm and peaceful surroundings, but please don't blame yourself for your baby's discomfort. A couple of our kids always had a fussy time in the evening, so we began to refer to it jokingly as "the sunset blues." In fact, keeping a sense of humor was our most important remedy. There is no foolproof method for preventing fussiness, but the following suggestions often help:

- ❧ Many babies get upset after their nursing moms have eaten a member of the cabbage family (broccoli, cabbage, kale, collards), turnips, garlic, onions, or spicy foods. Fried foods, peanuts, caffeine, dairy, eggs, beans, and wheat also may be aggravating. Avoid them while you are nursing.

- ❧ Hold your baby closely and firmly when you nurse, but don't fidget or distract the baby while he's eating. Nurse in quiet surroundings whenever possible. This will help prevent indigestion.

- ❧ Mother's Milk Blend II (see page 154) helps ease colic when taken by either mom or child and is also useful with hyperactivity, sleeplessness, and fussiness.

MOTHER'S MILK BLEND II

A few teaspoons of this tea, unsweetened (honey is not safe for children under 1 year), can be given directly to the baby.

1 ounce catnip leaves

1 ounce chamomile flowers

1 ounce lemon balm leaves

$1/2$ ounce fennel seeds

$1/4$ ounce of lavender flowers

Mix together all of the herbs. Store in a glass jar. When ready to use, place 2 tablespoons of the mix in a cup of boiling water. Steep, covered, for 15 minutes. Strain, sweeten if desired, and drink while still warm. Breathe in the sweet, soothing scent as you drink.

- Dill, caraway, and aniseed teas are useful for treating colic.

- If your baby has a regular fussy time, try to drink the tea before then. If possible, rest and eat well so you have the reserves you need to care for your baby without becoming frazzled.

- Bach Rescue Remedy, a flower essence, is a highly recommended item in the fussy-child repertoire. Give 2 drops to baby and 4 drops each to mother and father.

- Exercise the baby's legs by "bicycling" them, together and alternately, up to the baby's abdomen. Press the legs up to the belly (both, then individually), then extend them back out and down. Do each motion 5 times slowly and smoothly.

- Put your baby in a baby sling and go for a walk. The closeness your baby will feel with you, combined with the rocking motions of your body, may soothe her and help her settle down. The outdoors itself has a soothing influence on both baby and you.

When followed by a warm bath, these techniques can form the basis of what could become a pleasant family ritual. With luck, the baby may even fall asleep. Bear in mind the saying, "This too shall pass." You won't always be able to take away your baby's suffering, but you can be there giving love and extending a soothing hand.

INFANT MASSAGE

Infant massage is practiced in cultures all over the world, and is typically done by the mother of the baby, although sometimes a grandma does it.

Nowadays we have classes in infant massage, which can be a good way to meet other mothers while you learn massage techniques, but you don't have to take lessons to be good at massaging your baby. An excellent book full of techniques and stories is called *Infant Massage*, by Vimala McClure Schneider. Infant massage is a lovely way to relax for you and baby, and creates a special and intimate bond of touch between you. Furthermore, babies thrive on touch—regular massage is an excellent way to enhance growth, ensure optimal nervous system development, and promote immune health. It can also be used to soothe a fretful baby and reduce colic. Infant massage can be given several times a week, and is a perfect follow-up to baby's bath.

As our children grew, we continued to give them massage once a week. They still ask us to rub their feet before bed, and love to receive a massage when they are feeling unwell or have aches or pains.

Here's what to do. Place a soft cloth, towel, or mat in front of the mother in a warm room. Rub the baby with oil (coconut oil, almond oil, and cocoa butter are all excellent choices, but avoid scented oils, which might irritate a baby's sensitive skin). Rub the baby's abdomen with warm hands and a bit of the oil, using circular motions in a clockwise direction. Do this for 15 minutes slowly and gently, talking or singing to your baby as you rub. Another massage technique is to rub gently in a downward motion from beneath the ribs to the lower abdomen, using the pinkie-finger side of your hands. Alternate your hands continually so it looks like you are making a waterwheel motion on your baby's belly.

COPING WITH SLEEP DEPRIVATION

I've often said that mothers sleep with one eye open. Even when you're getting sleep, there is some part of you that's alert to the slightest signal that your baby needs you. This reflex allows you to be aware of your baby's needs, but can also lead to chronic tiredness. Mothers are always "on." Unfortunately, being short on sleep can mean being short on patience and long on tension. Find ways to get rest and extra sleep—you'll enjoy motherhood much more than if you're always exhausted. Sleeping with your baby on your chest can be a highly spiritual experience, as you and your baby melt into the connectedness you had during pregnancy, and this allows you to get deep rest while your baby sleeps. Occasionally let your partner cuddle with the baby in another room, while you take an afternoon nap with complete relaxation. Knowing your baby is well cared for will help you to sleep without continually waking to check on her, a common thing to do during the first couple of weeks after the birth.

⅔∽ SLEEPING ARRANGEMENTS ∞ⅇ

The idea of sleeping in the same bed with baby is very controversial in the United States, although this practice is common around the world. Misconceptions abound, including the notion that it is sexually inappropriate to have the child in the parents' bed, and that it is dangerous because the parents might smother the baby in their sleep. However, parents who practice co-sleeping or "family bed," particularly when their children are babies, find many advantages with this arrangement. The sense of connection between the mother and the baby is strongly maintained—the baby, having slept in Mom's belly for 9 months, can continue to benefit from the warmth of her skin and the sounds of her heartbeat and breathing. The baby is also stimulated by the mother's movements and sounds, which some researchers allege may actually lead to a reduction in SIDS.

Furthermore, it is more convenient for the mother who is breast-feeding to have baby in bed; she thus is able to nurse easily during the night without having to wake fully, get out of bed, feed the baby, and then put the baby back into his own bed. Whether to continue family bed past the first months or for a couple of years is a personal and individual choice, but for at least the first year, and again, especially for breast-feeding mothers, it's a nurturing and nourishing way for baby to sleep.

⅔∽ GETTING AROUND WITH BABY ∞ⅇ

There is so much unnecessary baby paraphernalia to choose from that one has to wonder how people ever managed to have babies before the invention of plastic. However, there are two seemingly indispensable baby-care items that do have their origins in traditional baby-care methods—baby slings and baby backpacks. Frankly, if it weren't for these devices, my life probably would have come to a grinding halt. After all, how do you cook a meal, work in the garden, or do much of anything with a baby in arms?

During the first few months after birth, until your baby is capable of holding her head up fairly well and for a long time, you can't use a metal-frame backpack. But you can use an over-the-shoulder sling, keeping one hand completely free and the other, with some skill and practice, almost completely free; or you can use a cloth front pack. The best cloth front packs can also be used on the back, enabling you to have both hands free and not bump the baby into the kitchen sink or stove while washing dishes or cooking a meal. Both front packs and slings are easy to put on without help, and both allow you to nurse the baby in the carrier. Cloth back carriers require some dexterity and practice to get the baby in alone, but it can be done. However, you have to take the baby out every time you need to nurse her. Fortunately, most babies will sleep in a pack for long periods, rocked by the movements of your body as you go about your work.

Eventually the baby will outgrow both the size and the confinement of the cloth baby pack, but by 3 months you can begin to use a metal-frame backpack, putting small firm pillows next to the baby to fill up the space and to prop her up. Before long, she'll be a steady backpack traveler. You can also continue to use the sling well for about 18 months. Choose a metal-frame backpack that distributes the weight over your hips as much as it does over your shoulders. Fancy sun visors and gadgets are just extras, but a couple of deep pockets enable you to get around with baby, a few diapers, and other necessities without also having to carry a diaper bag. Quite convenient!

I have to admit, as active as I am, my kids practically lived in backpacks. In fact, they've attended a number of births with me in my capacity as midwife, riding along on my shoulder, generally sound asleep, but occasionally there to witness the beginning of a new life—some of them children they have grown up with as friends!

❧ MORE EXERCISES FOR LOVING ☙ YOUR POST-BIRTH BODY

By now you are probably ready to achieve some level of exercise and activity, particularly if you were athletic and active before pregnancy and birth. You may also be ready to take a proactive role in regaining a semblance of your before-baby body shape. After 3 weeks postpartum you can begin gentle stretching exercises and take increasingly long walks, starting slowly and working up to more vigorous activity over several weeks.

Moderate yoga is fine now, but you should not do any inversion exercises such as headstands and shoulder stands until your bleeding has completely stopped. Similarly, you can begin light aerobics after 3 to 4 weeks postpartum, taking care to avoid heavy jumping and pounding movements.

At home, practice lunges and semi-squats to tone and shape the inner and outer thighs and buttocks, and modified sit-ups and mini crunches to wake up abdominal muscles. Forgo abdominal crunches if your rectus abdominus muscles have separated, a common result of the abdominal muscles stretching during pregnancy. Your midwife or obstetrician can tell you if they have separated, and can show you exercises to help restore their tone and position. Try some light workouts with arm weights (5 pounds) to strengthen and shape the arms.

If time to exercise is an issue, find creative ways to incorporate baby into your routine, such as putting the baby in a pack while you walk, or even using your baby as a weight—for example, lying on your back and lifting baby up and down over your chest. (*Warning:* Put a receiving blanket on your chest so you don't have to wear spit-up for the rest of the workout!)

If you want to undertake a new exercise routine, such as a dance class, wait until the baby is 4 to 6 weeks old. Let your instructor know you've just had a baby, and take it slowly at first. Drink plenty of water before, during, and after your workout, and make sure you're eating enough to compensate for calories lost during exercise, especially if you're nursing. You know your physical comfort—let it be your guide and don't push past your limits. Build up stamina, skill, or strength slowly.

Also, pay attention to your bleeding. If you had finished postpartum bleeding only to resume it once you began to exercise, unless it is your menstrual cycle returning you have done too much too fast. Slow down and be patient—slow and steady wins the race!

❧ BACK IN THE SWING ❧ OF THINGS

No matter how long you had help during the few weeks after the birth, it may feel like you didn't have enough. Even when my husband took 3 weeks off from work to care for our older children and me after our third and fourth babies were born, I always felt I could use another week or 10 of having him around full time. Yet a day must come when you and baby go it alone. It is common for new mothers to have anxieties about whether they can cope with baby and still meet their household responsibilities. It is also common for new moms to feel they can handle everything, only to disover that integrating baby into their life and still having time to meet their own basic needs is harder than they thought it would be.

It is important to remember that postpartum recovery length varies greatly. Some women feel great after a few days; others take weeks or even months to get back into the flow of their daily life. Most women find they fatigue more easily than before, and for some women discomforts such as a sore episiotomy site can have a serious impact on freedom of movement and even their emotional state. Breast-feeding moms may get hungry quickly, and somewhat insidiously, finding themselves in a blood-sugar crash before they realize they need to eat.

Mini breakdowns are common and to be expected—moments (or hours) of weeping or sobbing for no reason (or for good reason), utter exhaustion, or a sense of being totally overwhelmed. While these feelings cannot be entirely prevented, keeping up with good nutrition, drinking plenty of fluids, and getting lots of rest will certainly minimize the frequency and severity of these moments. Patience with yourself is also essential.

In the first few weeks after birth you've probably felt your priorities begin to shift (if they hadn't already during the pregnancy). If you are planning to go back to a job outside the home in several weeks, you may feel strong emotions ranging from excitement mixed with guilt if you want to return to your work, to all-out resentment and anxiety if you would prefer to stay home. Interestingly, you may have thought you'd want to return to your job, only to find yourself so engrossed with baby that you now want to be home full time. Just the opposite could also occur—being someone who thought you'd want to be home as a full-time mother, you discover you really want some time out of the house to be your professional self. Although many women do not have the luxury of choosing to stay home, all mothers who have had careers outside the home must face important and serious decisions after a baby is born. And while you may have a plan during the pregnancy, it is only after the baby is born and with you for a while that you can begin to develop a sense of what is right for you and the baby. Thus, it is ideal if you can keep your options open and plan for a variety of contingencies with your employer.

Regardless of whether you choose to remain home full time or return to your job in some capacity, you may feel so consumed by your daily life and so focused on your relationship with baby that you neglect your own social relationships or activities. It is perfectly normal to desire to be home-centered and focused on the baby, but it is very important to avoid becoming emotionally isolated. Make time to talk with friends or relatives, and after the first months, make sure you plan nurturing visits. At some point toward the end of your first 6 weeks, consider joining a mothers group if your friends, neighbors, or colleagues don't have children. You'll welcome being with other adults with whom you can share your ups and downs and get feedback, and will form relationships that help you feel normal and affirmed as you go through the myriad changes that parenthood brings.

⟿ WORKING AND BREAST FEEDING ⟾

It's true that every mother is a working mother. Both stay-at-home moms and those with jobs outside the home face challenges of time, personal satisfaction, and ability to manage multiple tasks. However, when it comes to breast feeding, mothers who leave home to work face challenges not encountered by those whose babies have continuous ready access to mom's breast. Fortunately, breast feeding has reemerged as an acceptable way to feed baby, and there are increasing numbers of women who have successfully navigated the job world while continuing to fully or partially breast feed. Unfortunately, federal work policies have not been established that promote and support breast feeding on the job, and many working mothers feel compromised in how fully they are able to nurse their babies.

There are as many good reasons to breast-feed your baby while working as there are good reasons to breast-feed, and immunologically, if your baby will be in childcare because you work, breast feeding is doubly important. Breast-fed babies get sick less often than do formula-fed babies. This means fewer sick days for you at work—a definite employer advantage. Breast feeding meets your baby's emotional needs for as long as the relationship continues, helping you to have a strong bond, even though you may face many hours of separation each day. Breast feeding gives you a sense of satisfaction that you can feed your baby and provide optimal nutrition each day, even if you can't provide the quantity of time you'd like to with your baby. Breast feeding is less expensive than formula feeding. Furthermore, breast feeding can save millions of dollars annually on medical bills nationally, due to reduction in rates of medical expenses, and employees save in reduced turnover, less absenteeism, and improved worker morale. Indeed, according to the Mother-Friendly Workplace Initiative Action Folder, some programs that support employee breast feeding have had a twofold return on money invested.

As early as 1919, the International Labor Organization (ILO) outlined measures to protect breast-feeding women in industry and commerce. These measures were revised in 1952, and set the following standards:

- 12 weeks maternity leave, 6 weeks before and 6 weeks after birth, with cash benefits of at least 66 percent of previous earnings;

- Two half-hour breast-feeding breaks during each working day; and

❧ Prohibition of dismissal during maternity leave.

Subsequent conventions of the ILO led to recommendations including increased benefits to working women and suggested paternal leave to aid employees with families.

The Mother-Friendly Workplace Initiative, much like the Baby-Friendly Hospital Initiative, promotes the benefits of creating workplaces that encourage and support breast feeding. The initiative targets three essential requirements for a mother-friendly workplace: time, space/proximity, and support.

MOTHER-FRIENDLY WORKPLACE INITIATIVE
Essential Components of a Mother-Friendly Workplace

Time

1. Provide at least four months paid maternity leave (with an ideal of six months) that begins after the baby is born. Offer other options such as longer maternity leave with partial pay.

2. Offer flexible work hours to breast-feeding women such as part-time schedules, longer lunch breaks, and job sharing.

3. Provide breast-feeding breaks of at least an hour a day.

Space/Proximity

1. Support infant and childcare at or near the workplace, and provide transportation for mothers to join their babies. For rural worksites and seasonal work, use mobile childcare units.

2. Provide comfortable, private facilities for expressing and storing breastmilk.

3. Keep the work environment clean and safe from hazardous wastes and chemicals.

Support

1. Inform women workers and unions about maternity benefits and provide information to support women's health.

2. Ensure that mothers have full job security.

3. Encourage co-workers and management to have a positive attitude toward breast feeding in public.

4. Encourage a network of supportive women in unions or worker's groups who can help women to combine breast-feeding and work.

WORKING MOTHERS CAN BREAST-FEED!

The Mother-Friendly Initiative gives the following tips for successful breast feeding while working:

- ❧ Take as much leave as possible after birth.

- ❧ Eat and drink extra to maintain your health. Make sure your diet is well balanced and includes lots of locally available fruits, vegetables, carbohydrates, and fluids.

- ❧ Get breast-feeding well established before returning to your job.

- ❧ If you will be away from your baby for several hours, express milk at similar times you would breast-feed in order to maintain the demand on your body and to allow your childcare provider to feed the baby with your milk.

- ❧ Be sure your childcare provider understands and supports breast feeding.

- ❧ Practice expressing milk before you return to work.

- ❧ Get extra help from family and friends while you are breast-feeding.

- ❧ Breast-feed in a comfortable position so you get some rest at the same time.

- ❧ Breast-feed more at night if you are separated from the baby a lot during the day. This is easier if the baby sleeps with you.

- ❧ If you have flexible hours, go in an hour late, extend your lunch break, or leave an hour early to maximize your time to breast-feed.

- ❧ Consider sharing childcare with another mother, or other methods of cooperative support with other mothers.

- ❧ Postpone your next pregnancy until you are ready to breast-feed another child.

Adapted from Women, Work, and Breastfeeding: Mother-Friendly Workplace Initiative Action Folder

As we have seen, economics don't have to be a factor in whether employed mothers can successfully breast-feed. However, it will take more pressure from more breast-feeding mothers to institute broad-scale social changes in the workplace. We also need more family-centered work and childcare models so that more women can work from home or near their babies, or at least have family they can rely on to help them out with baby.

❧ BREAST PUMPS, NURSING, ⚘ AND MAKING IT WORK

There are a number of excellent books that address the topic of work and breast feeding, so here I will cover only the basic points. I encourage you to read *The Breastfeeding Book,* by Martha and William Sears; *Nursing Mother, Working Mother,* by Gale Pryor; and *The Nursing Mother's Companion,* by Kathleen Huggins (see Bibliography). And remember to make use of La Leche League for local support and advice on working and nursing.

A key to successful milk expression is a well-established milk supply. Here are some tips for establishing a good milk supply:

- ❧ Nurse your baby often and for long periods. The more the baby nurses, the more milk you will have. Every 2 hours is perfectly reasonable.

- ❧ Nurse as often as the baby wants to and for as long as the baby wants to.

- ❧ Nurse at night, too.

- ❧ Eat well and drink plenty of fluids.

- ❧ Don't try to diet or lose weight quickly—this will affect your milk supply.

- ❧ Breast-feed and express milk in a relaxed environment to maximize the let-down reflex.

- ❧ Allow your baby to stay on one side for each feeding. At a long feeding, switch after 20 to 30 minutes at each breast. Switching every 10 minutes, as is often advised, can be painful for you, and also doesn't allow the baby to reach the rich hind milk or to empty the breast. Alternate sides with each feeding.

Expressing milk is easier for some women than others, even if they have the same abundance of milk. A big factor in successful pumping may be the let-down or milk-ejection reflex. To encourage your milk to let down, hand-express or pump in a relaxed environment and think about your baby, or at least have your baby nearby. Some women prefer and have better results with manual expression, but most prefer a hand or electric pump. Medela (see Resources) makes excellent pumps that you can rent or purchase. Be gentle as you learn to express so you don't irritate or bruise your nipples. Your midwife, a La Leche League Leader, or a lactation consultant can teach you how to effectively express milk.

✤ RELATIONSHIP CHALLENGES ✤
AND TRIUMPHS

The postpartum time may put relationships to the test, as emotions are raw and the concept of sleep deprivation achieves new meaning. Your needs may be strong, and you are probably experiencing a range of emotional highs and lows, sometimes shifting from one to another with little notice. If you and your partner have seasoned your friendship and your ability to communicate and understand each other with patience, this can be a very rich time. It can also be a trying time. Postpartum brings with it a lot of earthy realities that you and your mate might not have previously faced with each other. After all, having your partner tend to your perineum or hemorrhoids is not the stuff of romance, nor are leaking breasts when you make love, baby vomit on your pajamas, or any of the other daily joys you encounter as new parents.

Furthermore, you may focus so intently on baby that your mate feels insecure, resentful, displaced, overlooked, ignored, or all of these put together. You may feel "touched out" and exhausted, wanting only to collapse into yourself at the end of the day (or the middle of a weekend afternoon!). A husband may feel overwhelmed or confused by his partner's needs and emotions, and not know how to meet them. And even though he may genuinely want to support you full time and 100 percent, he may not have time flexibility at work.

External demands and conflicting pressures can cause tension between you even though you love each other and want to be there for each other. The stresses of postpartum might persist for some time, as you adjust to new roles and demands, and have less time for each other and your relationship.

It will be helpful if you remember that fathers need nurturing, too. Even if you can't give out anymore yourself, acknowledge to your husband that you recognize he is going through a lot of changes and has a lot of pressures—this will help him feel less stressed. It can also be helpful if you set aside some time each week, or at least every 2 weeks, to nurture your personal relationship, friendship, and intimacy (even in nonsexual ways). Take an hour to recite your wedding vows to each other; to take a bath together with baby asleep or in a safe place nearby; to read poetry or watch a movie; to enjoy a cup of tea and dessert by candlelight. Frequently, even a little focused time put into a relationship goes a long way.

❧ SEX IN THE WEEKS AFTER BIRTH ❧

Few women want to make love in the first weeks after birth. Midwives and others suggest you wait until your postpartum bleeding has stopped and until you are completely ready—physically and emotionally—to resume sexual activity. Some women who have had an uncomplicated birth and neither perineal tears nor an episiotomy are ready to resume having sex 4 to 6 weeks postpartum, but many women, especially those who have had some perineal trauma, prefer not to have sex, especially intercourse, for several months after birth.

Although this may be difficult for your partner to understand, it is perfectly normal. In fact, several studies reveal that postpartum sexual tensions are very common, with 20 percent of all women not resuming intercourse until after 3 months postpartum. Women who breast-fed their babies, whether due to hormonal reasons, fatigue, or simply having had enough of being touched each day, were significantly less interested in resuming sexual activity. Some breast-feeding mothers are just so satisfied with their relationship with the baby that sex is not a high need for them.

Women who have experienced a difficult birth, especially with an accompanying sense of physical invasion, may have deep resentments and grief that are triggered by sexual physical intimacy.

All this can be very challenging to your partner to understand, and he may be impatient to make love with you, especially if he has already gone many months at the end of the pregnancy with you not wanting to have sex. Also, your partner may be very turned on by watching you nurture and breast-feed the baby, so your lack of interest may be further frustrating to him, and he may feel jealous of the attention you shower on your little one.

This is a time for patience and sensitivity from both of you. Find ways to understand each other's needs and gently and creatively meet them—this can prevent tension from building up in your marriage, and both of you will reap the rewards. Try to find ways to bring your partner pleasure that don't infringe on your need to wait to resume an active sexual relationship. If you don't want to make love yet, your partner will have to respect this.

If trauma at the birth, either emotionally or physically, has left you feeling vulnerable or uncomfortable, or if you have fears about resuming sex, talk to your childbirth provider, who can evaluate you physically and allay your fears; or talk to a birth counselor to help resolve your negative feelings.

If you are ready to resume sexual activity, even within the first few weeks postpartum, check with your midwife or other care provider to make sure any tears or small abrasions (midwives refer to these as "skid marks") are healed. Many breast-feeding mothers don't have much vaginal lubrication. Reassure your mate that it is not lack of interest, just breast feeding, that is preventing you from being moist. A nice vaginal cream, oil lubricant, or KY jelly provides moisture. Remember, you can get pregnant again even in the first couple of months after giving birth, so speak with your care provider about birth-control options during the postpartum. Your partner can use a condom (oil lubricants can break down latex, so don't use these together), as before, but if you had a diaphragm or cervical cap, you must be refitted for size.

❧ *Gentle Vaginal Lubricant*

Sandalwood and vanilla together are a highly aphrodisiac scent.

> 4 tablespoons cocoa butter
> 4 tablespoons coconut oil
> 2 tablespoons almond oil
> 10 drops sandalwood essential oil
> 10 drops vanilla essential oil

Combine all ingredients, store in a jar, and apply as needed.

❧ BABY BLUES ❧

Every woman who has been pregnant, given birth, and been through the postpartum will tell you there is a huge range of emotions, from the happiest to the most desperate, that you go through in the course of becoming a mother. Most women, in the days, weeks, and months after birth, will go through moments—or longer—of extremes of emotion. This is normal and to be expected. You are experiencing a lot right now—love, vulnerability, adjustment, exhaustion, healing, discomfort, insecurity, triumph, and enormous hormonal and physical changes. This is profound time of openness and depth of feeling, often accompanied by a sense of lack of control: over your body, your baby, your time. For a variety of reasons, from hormonal causes to psychosocial influences, a small percentage of women will experience the depths of the more painful and difficult of these emotions, sometimes for months at a time. The emotions women may experience can be classified on a continuum ranging from momentary feelings of sadness, to baby blues, to postpartum depression. A rare and extreme form of severe postpartum depression is known as postpartum psychosis.

Occasionally I get a client in my midwifery practice who remembers stories of a family member—a grandmother, great-aunt, or perhaps even her own mom if the client is in her 40s or older—who was institutionalized after becoming a mother. This was the common treatment, until not long ago, for extreme depression after birth. Now postpartum depression is recognized as a treatable syndrome in its own right. Such stories can have a haunting effect on a new mother—or on a new father if he has heard stories from his own family and is afraid of this happening to his wife. Fortunately for women now, postpartum depression is considered "100 percent treatable" (Placksin 2000).

Periods of weepiness, anxiety, and irritability that generally occur between 3 and 10 days after birth describe the baby blues. They last from several hours to several days. Studies indicate that 30 to 80 percent of all women will experience the baby blues. The feeling is attributed primarily to the significant drop in hormones that occurs after birth. It is aggravated by fatigue and low blood sugar. Feelings of disappointment about the birth, or lack of support in the postpartum, also contribute to the baby blues. The best treatment for baby blues is to express your feelings, ask for more support, get plenty of rest, especially when the baby rests, eat well, and drink plenty of fluids. Make sure you keep up your prenatal vitamins. Relaxing herbs might be helpful to take the edge off jangled nerves. Consider the following tincture blend (see pages 242–44 for more about tinctures):

 Mother's Nerve Support
$1/2$ ounce motherwort tincture
$1/2$ ounce vitex (chaste tree) tincture
$1/4$ ounce lavender tincture
$1/4$ ounce lemon balm tincture
$1/4$ ounce passionflower tincture
$1/4$ ounce skullcap tincture

Combine all of these ingredients into one blend.
Dose: Take $1/2$ to 1 teaspoon as needed, up to 4 teaspoons daily for 2 weeks

Remember, "All women—and parents—go through a profound adjustment after the birth of a baby. In part, the extent to which a new mom is permitted to express her real feelings in a non-judgmental atmosphere may affect the ease or difficulty of her adjustment" (Placksin). Yes, there are profound physical and chemical changes that lead to baby blues, but don't just write off your feelings as "hormonal"—express them, get support, and treat yourself like the queen you deserve to be as you adjust to your new role as mother.

ᴖᴗ POSTPARTUM DEPRESSION ᴖᴗ

*Women are the experts of their own lives, yet their voices are
missing in the existing body of knowledge about depression
after childbirth.*

**K. Berggren-Klive, "Out of the Darkness and Into the Light:
Women's Experiences with Depression After Childbirth,"
in *Canadian Journal of Community Mental Health*, 1998**

Postpartum depression (PPD) is thought to affect between 4 and 28 percent of all mothers. Despite its prevalence, it is not well understood. PPD can occur anytime in the first year postpartum, but may be prolonged beyond this time. Breast-feeding mothers may be significantly less likely to develop postpartum depression (Abou-Saleh et al. 1998). Symptoms of PPD include irritability, guilt, hopelessness, despair, insomnia, difficulty concentrating, confusion, inability to cope, thoughts of hurting oneself or baby (see the following chart for a complete list). It is the duration, severity, and complexity of the symptoms that distinguish postpartum depression from the baby blues. Few women experience all of these symptoms.

Women with postpartum depression may also be consumed by the terrible feeling that they will always be this way—that the depression and anxiety will never go away. They may feel extremely detached from their family, including their husband, baby, and other children. It can be terrifying for women to feel this way and not to know when, if ever, this will end. They may also be horrified at their thoughts of hurting the baby. This can cause panic and anxiety, leading them to distance themselves from the baby and exacerbating feelings of inadequacy as a mother. For most women, an actual diagnosis of postpartum depression is a tremendous relief—it places their experience into the context of an illness for which there is a treatment and cure, and which will eventually end. It provides a framework that helps them, as well as their family, begin to make sense of what is happening.

Too often, postpartum depression is dismissed as "just the baby blues," leaving women who need treatment and care with none and prolonging the terrible desperation they feel. It is often women who did not receive adequate support in the first place who develop severe PPD, so seeking help becomes all the more critical for these women. Even help as simple as talking with a therapist can lead to significant improvement in PPD. In one study, interpersonal psychotherapy was demonstrated to reduce depressive symptoms and improve adjustment, and was shown to be an alternative to drug therapy, especially for breast-feeding mothers (O'Hara et al. 2000). It is important for women who are experiencing extreme or prolonged symptoms to seek help.

SYMPTOMS OF POSTPARTUM DEPRESSION

agitation

anxiety or panic attacks

chronic exhaustion

clumsiness

confusion

decreased appetite or extreme cravings

depression

despair

difficulty relaxing or concentrating

emotional numbness

fear

feelings of inadequacy

frequent crying or inability to cry

guilt

hopelessness

inability to cope

inability to function

insomnia

irrational overconcern with baby's well-being

irritability

joylessness

lack of attention to appearance

loneliness

loss of normal interests

memory loss

mood swings

nightmares

thoughts of hurting oneself or baby

withdrawal from social contacts

Note: Experiencing some of these symptoms does not mean you have PPD. If you have severe symptoms, many of these symptoms, or persistent symptoms, speak with your midwife or care provider.

There is still stigma attached to depression, so too many people who need help avoid getting it. Fortunately, there is a greater understanding and sensitivity about postpartum depression than ever before. There are more treatment options as well, and with the widespread marketing of drugs such as Prozac and Zoloft, depression in general has come out of the closet, making it easier for women to admit to the illness and seek help.

The biggest problem in the treatment of postpartum depression is the uncertainty about causative factors. Most often in the medical literature and in the minds of physicians, PPD is attributed to hormonal changes after birth and other biochemical origins such as thyroid deficiency (hypothyroidism), which is commonly found in the 2 to 5 months after birth. It is also frequently attributed to a "tendency to depression" (Small et al. 1997).

Women, however, are more likely to consider a "wide range of social, physical health, and life event factors as contributing to their experience of depression" (Small et al. 1997). One study, conducted in Switzerland, confirms women's beliefs on the origins of PPD. It found that among the most significant risk factors for postpartum depression are social or professional difficulties, deleterious life events, early mother-child separation, and negative birth experience (Righetti-Veltema et al. 1998). Another study cites poor support with newborn care as a factor in PPD, with affiliation with a secular group to be a positive preventative (Dankner et al. 2000). A study looking at the impact of a supportive partner in the treatment of PPD found a significant decrease in depressive symptoms in the group in which the partner provided the mother with significant support. Yet another study indicated that women with postpartum depression "reported less practical and emotional support from their partners and saw themselves as having less social support overall" (Small et al. 1994). Clearly, adequate social support is an important variable in preventing postpartum depression.

DID YOU KNOW . . .

Some 400,000 women each year suffer from postpartum depression.

The birth experience itself may have a dramatic impact on a woman's view of herself and her postpartum recovery or tendency to depression, yet this factor is generally overlooked. One study indicates that assisted delivery (cesarean, forceps, and vacuum extraction) were associated with higher rates of postnatal depression, as were bottle-feeding, dissatisfaction with prenatal care, having unwanted people present at the birth, and lack of confidence to care for the baby after they left the hospital (Astbury et al. 1994). A study by Edwards et al. (1994) indicates a significant increase in rates of postpartum depression among women who have had cesarean sections. Considering that 25 percent of American women now deliver by C-section, this illuminates the need to both reduce cesarean rates and provide counseling and support for those women who have birthed operatively. The need for women to have excellent support before birth and during labor to help encourage a natural and smooth birth experience without intervention whenever possible is evident. Furthermore, one study indicates that women who were cared for by midwives had lower rates of depression in the postnatal period (Shields et al. 1997), while another study revealed a significantly lower rate of depression among the women who gave birth at home compared to hospital vaginal delivery (Shields et al. 1997). Women reported that a sense of control and being informed about choices in their healthcare greatly improved their psychological state.

Nutrition can also play a part in postpartum depression, particularly regarding the need for essential fatty acids, protein, B vitamins, zinc, and iron. Women who have experienced significant blood loss at birth may be predisposed to depression due to anemia and its accompanying increased fatigue and tendency to infection. Low blood sugar can have a dramatic effect on mood; therefore, postpartum women must ensure adequate caloric intake through a well-balanced diet to minimize the risk of depression due to hypoglycemia.

PLAY IT SAFE

If you are experiencing extreme depression, suicidal thoughts, or thoughts of harming your baby, please seek professional help. This is nothing to be ashamed of. Early identification and treatment of postpartum depression can decrease the duration of the condition and dramatically improve your sense of well-being.

If you suspect your wife or a friend of having postpartum depression, help her find help. If you think you or a loved one is in crisis with PPD, seek help immediately through an emergency hotline or the local emergency room. To connect with a local support group or counselor, contact:

Postpartum Support, International (California) 805-967-7636

Because hotline numbers change regularly, visit its Web site for the contact nearest you: www.postpartum.net

Many people are afraid to talk to women about postpartum depression during the prenatal period. Much like their hesitation to discuss complications of birth during pregnancy, they think it might create negative thinking or frighten a mother-to-be. This, however, is far from the truth; in fact, a woman will be better prepared to recognize her need for help and get it if she is informed ahead of time that this could happen. According to Jane Honikman, founder of Postpartum Support, International, as quoted in Placksin, "Ignorance and denial are the two greatest barriers to this problem."

Talking about postpartum depression before birth can actually have a positive impact in reducing depression because it will help a mother develop realistic goals and expectations for herself. Many women enter pregnancy with an unrealistic picture of motherhood.

There are also tremendous social pressures on women to conform to the image of being happy and grateful (Placksin). In fact, social pressures strongly contribute to women's sense of inadequacy—leaving them feeling that "everyone else does better than I do and is happy, why can't I be?" It is essential that women speak out, support each other, and be honest about the joys and difficulties of mothering. It is hard to fully enjoy an experience that is laden with stress and anxiety. Women need to know that while these feelings are common, they need not materialize. We should not be burdened by lack of support, depression, anxiety, and loneliness when we enter motherhood. We should do so with celebration. Perhaps in the honesty and revelations women have that they are not alone and not crazy, and that they are good mothers, will actually emerge a renewed enjoyment for motherhood.

START YOUR OWN NETWORK

If you want to set up a postpartum support network in your community, get a copy of *Step by Step: A Guide for Organizing a Parent Postpartum Group*, by Jane Honikman, available through Postpartum Support, International (see Resources).

TREATING POSTPARTUM DEPRESSION

In her excellent book *Mothering the New Mother*, Sally Placksin quotes the work of medical anthropologist Dr. Laurence Kruckman, who has studied postpartum traditions in many cultures. Kruckman concludes that "where there was support for the new mom, including rites of passage and healing ceremonies, there was also . . . a cushioning effect that helped ease her adjustment through this transitional time in her life." In our society, women receive no such rites or ceremonies after birth, and are pretty much left to their own devices to care for their families. Perhaps one of the most important factors in both preventing and treating women with postpartum depression is to rally around new moms with abundant and generous support. In addition, women with postpartum depression can seek the emotional support of counselors who are trained to help them cope and come out on the other side.

Extreme treatments such as hospitalization are rarely necessary; however, pharmacotherapy in the form of antidepressant drugs, hormonal therapies, or medications to aid sleep is commonly prescribed. Drug therapy lasts only for the duration of the condition, which is not permanent. Medications can be helpful, but most women would prefer not to take them when caring for a baby. This is a very personal decision and should be based on an assessment of the risks and benefits of any kind of drug therapy. If you are nursing, your doctor will try to prescribe something that can be taken safely while breast-feeding. If the medication requires you to discontinue breast feeding and you think that will only add to your depression, be sure to tell your doctor and see if he can modify your program to enable you to continue to nurse.

Alternative therapies often constitute effective treatment for mild to moderate depression, but should be undertaken with the guidance of a qualified healthcare provider and in conjunction with your physician if you are using medications. Nutritional and herbal therapies both have been shown to reduce depression in many cases. Nutritional therapies, mentioned earlier, include improving overall caloric intake through a well-balanced diet, increasing protein consumption, and ensuring adequate intake of vitamins and minerals through foods and supplemented with a prenatal vitamin. The addition of essential fatty acids in the form of either a fish-oil supplement or evening primrose oil (2,500 mg daily) can be helpful, as can a B-complex supplement. Inadequate fluid intake aggravates depression—be sure to get at least 2 liters of water each day. Avoid caffeine, chocolate, coffee, and sodas, and keep sugar consumption to a minimum.

HERBAL THERAPIES FOR PPD

Herbal remedies are the primary therapy for the treatment of depression in many European countries and are increasingly recognized in the United States as safe and effective alternatives to many psychotherapeutic medications. Unfortunately, little, if any, research has been done into the safety and efficacy of using these herbs for postpartum depression or even simply during lactation. The recommendations below are based on known safe clinical use from herbal practitioners, combined with known issues of herbal contraindication for nursing mothers. As with any therapy, use caution and common sense. If your condition persists or worsens in spite of herbal treatments, discontinue the herbs and seek medical advice.

Herbs can be used for a variety of aspects of PPD, including the treatment of depression itself, reduction of anxiety, improvement of sleep, in support of and to regulate hormones, and as general nerve tonics. The following sections categorize the actions. Listed in parentheses next to the herb is the form in which the herb is generally recommended. You can combine herbs from these categories, or choose from the sample formulas that follow.

Nervous System Relaxants

Blue vervain (tincture)
Chamomile (tea, tincture)
Lavender (tea, tincture)
Lemon balm (tea, tincture)
Linden (tea, tincture)

Milky oats (tincture, oats as food)
Motherwort (tincture)
Passionflower (tincture)
Skullcap (tincture)

Herbs to Reduce Anxiety

Chamomile (tea, tincture)
Kava kava (tincture)
Motherwort (tincture)
Passionflower (tincture)

St. John's wort (tincture)
Valerian (tincture)
Zizyphus (tea, tincture)

Nervous System Tonics

American ginseng (tincture)
Ashwaganda (tincture)
Blue vervain (tincture)
Eleuthero (tincture)

Ginseng (tea, soup, tincture)
Milky oats (tincture)
St. John's wort (tincture)

Antidepressants

Eleuthero (tincture)
Ginkgo (tincture)
Ginseng (tea, soup, tincture)

Kava kava (tincture)
Rosemary (tea, tincture)
St. John's wort (tincture)

Herbs to Promote Sleep

Chamomile (tea, tincture)

Hops (tincture)

Lavender (tea, tincture)

Passionflower (tincture)

Skullcap (tincture)

Hormonal Regulation

Dang gui (tea, soup, tincture)

Peony (tea, tincture)

Vitex (tincture)

Blood and General Tonics to Build Energy and Stamina

Dang gui (tea, soup, tincture)

Ginseng (tea, soup, tincture)

Licorice (tea, tincture)

Ligusticum (tea, tincture)

Nettle (tea, tincture, food)

Peony (tea, tincture)

Polygonum multiflorum (tea, tincture)

Rehmannia (tea, soup, tincture)

Schizandra (tincture)

Sample Formulas for Treating Postpartum Depression

These formulas can be used by nursing and nonnursing mothers for the treatment of postpartum depression. Or create your own formula by choosing herbs from the categories above and combining them to suit your specific needs.

 Tincture Formula 1

Simon Mills and Kerry Bone, in *Principals and Practice of Phytotherapy*, recommend this specifically for the treatment of PPD caused by hormonal effects and adrenal depletion. They recommend an additional 2 ml of vitex on rising each day.

> 30 ml ashwaganda
>
> 25 ml St. John's wort
>
> 20 ml blue vervain
>
> 15 ml licorice
>
> 10 ml ginseng

Dose: 5 ml (1 tsp.) with water, 3 times daily

 Tincture Formula 2

Use when anxiety and depression are the prominent symptoms, and for lack of mental clarity.

> 20 ml eleuthero

20 ml rosemary

20 ml St. John's wort

10 ml kava kava

10 ml licorice

10 ml motherwort

10 ml schizandra

10 ml vitex

Dose: 5 ml (1 tsp.) with water, 2 or 3 times daily

 ### Tincture Formula 3

For general irritability and weepiness.

25 ml blue vervain

25 ml motherwort

25 ml nettle

25 ml skullcap

Dose: 5 ml (1 tsp.) with water, 2 or 3 times daily

Tincture Formula 4

Primarily for insomnia and exhaustion related to insomnia.

30 ml passionflower

20 ml chamomile

20 ml linden

20 ml skullcap

10 ml lavender

Dose: 5 ml (1 tsp.) with water, 2 or 3 times daily, plus ¹/₂ teaspoon every 30 minutes for 2 hours before bed

THE LIGHT AT THE END OF THE TUNNEL

This chapter has been a long journey through the quickly passing but incredibly complex first 6 weeks after birth. By now many things have gotten easier for you, and you have enjoyed watching your baby blossom into a tiny little person with a distinct personality. This is a time of great joy and great challenge. In many ways you are through the steepest part of the learning curve and starting to settle into a family routine and the rest of your first postpartum year.

SIX

Nutrition for New Mothers

*Where you can cure by diet, use no drugs, and where simple
measures suffice, use no complex ones.*
Rhazes, father of Arabic medicine, Persia, A.D. 853–945

*D*uring pregnancy you have to be so extra-careful about your diet to
meet baby's nutritional needs that by the end of pregnancy you may
find that eating healthy has become a chore. Now baby is born and you're
ready to throw that careful diet out the window, but you still want to be
healthy, produce adequate breast milk, and maybe lose that 10 or 15 pounds
you still have from the pregnancy. Well, there is good news. You can eat properly, produce plenty of milk for your baby, lose weight, and still not have to
stress over diet. This chapter will explain what you need to eat and how to
keep it simple.

NOT PREGNANT ANYMORE: WHAT YOU NEED NOW

Pregnancy, though a process of great strength and power, also has the potential to take a lot from a woman's body. After all, it is truly your body that
builds that of your child, and nature has designed the process so that baby's
needs are met first. Therefore, it's the mother's nutrients that are depleted if
her diet does not adequately compensate for the demands of pregnancy.

Fortunately, nature in her infinite wisdom has also created some protective mechanisms for both baby and mother. For example, during pregnancy and breast feeding, calcium is spared through increased efficiency of
absorption and decreased excretion. Nonetheless, the increased caloric and
nutrient requirements of pregnancy and birth placed unique demands on
your body, and during the early postpartum it is important that you continue to eat a diet high in nutrients to promote healing, particularly if you

have had a surgical procedure at birth, including episiotomy or cesarean.

If you do not plan to breast-feed, your postnatal nutritional demands are not as high as if you do choose to nurse, but you must still eat a well-balanced, healthy diet to keep up with the increased demands of motherhood—including sleep loss, which is a natural part of the job description and can be stressful. A balanced diet is also the key to healthy weight loss after birth.

❧ LACTATION AND NUTRITION ❧

During pregnancy your body goes through changes to prepare for producing milk, including depositing body fat so you'll have reserves after the birth. Breast feeding adds to your postnatal nutrient demands. Breast-feeding moms actually need 500 to 700 calories more per day than do pregnant women. This is because the baby is growing faster than it did when in the womb, and because the baby is more active than a fetus. Newborns also have increased energy and nutrient needs for processes such as temperature regulation and digestion that were automatically managed by you before birth. Some of these calories are drawn from fat stores accumulated during pregnancy, a mechanism that ensures adequate calories even in the absence of adequate nutrition, and one of the reasons that breast feeding helps you to lose weight. During the first 6 months of breast-feeding, women produce on average 3 cups of milk daily, more or less according to how much the baby nurses. It takes about 225 calories to produce 1 cup of breast milk, which in turn provides the baby with approximately 175 calories. Fat stored during pregnancy will provide 200 to 300 calories daily for the first 3 months of breastfeeding. The rest must be derived from the mother's diet.

According to William and Martha Sears in *The Breastfeeding Book,* breast-feeding mothers need to eat a nutritious diet plus 20 percent more. This might seem overwhelming after your careful pregnancy diet, but at least you don't have to worry about whether your baby is getting enough of the right things—you can actually watch him grow. Also, by now food probably tastes good to you again if it didn't during pregnancy, so eating well can be a pleasure. It is important to remember that most women who breast-feed produce good-quality milk for their young, with the exception of those who suffer extreme nutritional deprivation. If you are reading this book, you probably don't have to worry about your milk quality or about becoming seriously depleted yourself. However, most of us want to feed our babies and ourselves optimally, not just adequately.

THE BREAST-FEEDING DIET

The optimal breast-feeding diet, like the best pregnancy diet, is full of nutrient-dense foods. These are those that contain a maximum amount of nutrition with a minimum of empty calories from sugar and fat. A yogurt smoothie made with fresh fruit is a nutrient-dense food loaded with protein, minerals, and vitamins; potato chips are empty calories, providing mostly fat and salt. Foods that are nutrient dense include yogurt, eggs, beans, tofu, fish, chicken, sweet potatoes, leafy green vegetables, vegetables in general, avocados, sunflower seeds, walnuts, almonds, peanut butter, butter, hard cheese, whole grains, and fresh fruits. It's simple to build your diet around these foods, as there are so many options.

However, having a newborn or young baby often means you have less time to prepare healthy foods for yourself—and for that matter, less time to eat them. I can remember in the early days of caring for my babies that food would go bad in the refrigerator just because it was too hard to prepare it or eat it with one hand! It is important that your breast-feeding diet be not only nutritious but also tasty and enjoyable. The last thing you need right now is increased stress, guilt, or pressure. Food should be as pleasurable for you as you want breast feeding to be for your baby. This requires a bit of planning and, in the beginning, a bit of help from your mate or other support people in your life.

TRADITIONAL CHINESE MEDICINE: RECIPES FOR NEW MOMS

Healing with foods is an important aspect of traditional Chinese medicine. The belief is that if healing can be done with food, this is the best medicine. Indeed, herbs are often put into foods to enhance nourishment and as a method of delivering the medicine in a pleasant, nutritive manner.

Traditional dietary practices often prove quite effective under scientific scrutiny. For example, studies show that 30 grams of soy protein can increase the volume of a mother's breast milk by as much as 25 percent (Sears and Sears 2000), and a study in the *European Journal of Clinical Nutrition* (Chan et al., 2000) demonstrated that "Ginger Vinegar Soup" has a higher level of calcium than six other soups. The iron level was also higher than that of other soups and was comparable to many iron-rich foods. According to this study, chicken soup was also commonly prescribed for postpartum and consumed by Hong Kong Chinese women after birth.

The following recipes were shared by Chinese herbalist Andy Ellis, himself the father of three. Although some of these recipes may seem unusual, they are considered excellent tonics for replenishing new mothers in the first week after birth.

 Peanut, Garlic, and Jujube Date Soup

This soup is said to "fortify the center" or nourish the *qi*, the vital energy of the body. It also moves stagnant energy and supplements the blood.

> 125 grams raw peanuts
> 30 grams fresh garlic
> 10 red jujube dates

Clean the peanuts and peel the skins off the garlic. Slice the garlic thinly and sauté in a small amount of vegetable oil. Add the peanuts, dates, and 4 cups of water. Simmer until the peanuts are soft.

Dose: Take $^1/_2$ cup, 4 times a day

 Mutton Stew with Dang Gui and Fresh Ginger

This stew nourishes the blood, reduces spasmodic pain, and warms the body. (This recipe is also found in *Chinese Herbal Medicine: Formulas and Strategies*, by Bensky and Barolett.)

> 2 ounces mutton
> 15 grams fresh gingerroot
> 9 grams dang gui
> 9 grams astragalus root (optional)

Prepare as a stew by simmering the mutton, gingerroot, and dang gui in 8 cups of water until reduced to 3 cups of liquid.

Dose: 2 or 3 servings of the liquid with the meat are all that is necessary. If you suffer from profuse postpartum sweating, add the astragalus root to the stew.

Note: I've seen several babies develop a small heat rash when the mother took dang gui during the first three months postpartum. This is not harmful and will disappear when you discontinue the use of the herb.

 Increase Breast Milk

Thought to nourish deficient blood and qi.

> 120 grams tofu
> 30 grams brown sugar
> 2 teaspoons yellow rice vinegar

Put the tofu and sugar in a medium saucepan. Add 3 cups of water, bring to a medium heat, and reduce to 2 cups, then add the rice wine vinegar.
Dose: $^1/_2$ cup 2 or 3 times daily

❧ PLANNING A HEALTHY DIET ❧

The first thing is to brainstorm a list of foods you like to eat. If you're short on ideas, pull out several of your favorite cookbooks, or purchase a couple of new ones and browse through them, jotting down some interesting recipes. Come up with a master list of easy-to-prepare, healthful foods that meet your postpartum nutritional needs. Foods that work well as leftovers for the next day get four stars! Post this list on the refrigerator, and when you need food ideas, turn to it.

Next, use that list to make a master shopping list, and ask someone to get the ingredients you need. Once your baby is several weeks old, you'll probably feel up to making a quick shopping trip, but let someone else lift heavy grocery bags. When you make your list, keep in mind things that are simple to heat and serve with one hand, particularly in the first 6 weeks after birth. Remember foods you might like to eat as snacks both during the day and at night before bed, as breast feeding will increase your appetite significantly. And keep in mind foods that are nutrient dense.

As life with a new baby is usually hectic, many women find it difficult to sit down for regular meals; instead they graze throughout the day. This is perfectly fine as long as you graze on high-quality, healthful foods. Calorie counting is unnecessary, as is counting other nutrients such as protein. Eat whenever you're hungry, and make what you eat nutritious. Because your life might be too busy for extensive cooking, stock the pantry with the ingredients you need for cooking quick meals, and plan ahead when you do cook so you have 2 or 3 days' worth of leftovers. You'll appreciate this foresight, as babies notoriously want to have their biggest nursing period just when you're ready to prepare supper!

DAILY FOOD CHOICES

Sometimes you get so caught up in caring for your baby or juggling a busy schedule that you scrimp on your own nutrition—or simply forget to eat—only to find yourself famished, irritable, or having other signs of a blood-sugar crash. This often happens after the baby has nursed fully—it is easy to overlook just how much energy nursing a baby and running a household require. Rather than getting so hungry that you reach for the nearest choco-late bar or bag of chips, be prepared.

The following list, based on the U.S. Department of Agriculture food pyramid for pregnancy and lactation, gives you a general idea of the number of food servings in various categories that you should strive to eat each day. In parentheses next to the lactation recommendation, I've put the pregnancy recommendations, just for comparison. Remember, you don't have to pre-pare three gourmet meals a day to meet your nutrient needs. Graze and snack as much as you need to; keep it simple and light. Just keep it healthy.

> Bread group: 10 servings daily (8)
> Vegetable group: 3 servings daily (3)
> Fruit group: 3 servings daily (3)
> Dairy group: 3 servings daily (3)
> Meat group: 7 ounces daily (6 oz)
> Fats, oils, and sweets: use sparingly

Vegetarian mothers should follow the same precautions for meeting their protein needs during lactation as they did during pregnancy, and women who use no dairy products (vegan) must also pay particular attention to cal-cium and vitamin B_{12} intake during lactation.

Protein

Protein needs are not increased from pregnancy to lactation, and, in fact, may be slightly less. Nonetheless, be sure to eat high-quality protein foods, including beans and legumes, tofu, nuts and seeds, lean meat, chicken, and fish as a regular part of your daily diet.

Carbohydrates

The healthiest forms of carbohydrates are complex carbohydrates, long chains of slow-burning sugars found in whole grains: whole wheat, brown rice, mil-let, buckwheat, barley, oats, and quinoa, among others. If you don't know how to cook whole grains, a trip to the bookstore or natural foods store will surely turn up a cookbook with excellent recipes and cooking suggestions. Whole grains provide energy, many vitamins, and plenty of fiber to keep digestion healthy. Pasta, too, is a good source of energy, and lends itself well to combinations with a wide variety of vegetables and healthful sauces.

Vitamins and Minerals

Getting several servings of fruits and vegetables daily, along with nuts, seeds, whole grains, and some dairy products, should provide ample nutrients for both you and baby. It's always best to derive your nutrients from food rather than relying on a supplement; however, during lactation a supplement can be beneficial, particularly if you are busy and not able to eat as well as you need to. Although breast feeding may deplete calcium stores initially, in the long run it may actually be beneficial for your bone density. Researchers have found that this initial calcium loss is only temporary, and that by the end of a year breast feeding is actually protective against bone loss and fractures because the body replaces what was used for making milk and then some with enhanced calcium uptake. Osteoporosis is actually less common in later life among women who have breast-fed.

Fats

Fat has become a bad word among the health conscious, due to its links with obesity and cardiovascular disease. However, some fats are actually beneficial for both you and the baby. Certain fats are an essential part of the diet and fat is the major component in breast milk, where it helps to promote the baby's brain growth and development. Indeed, good fats can actually reduce the risk of heart disease.

So which fats are healthy? Healthy fats are found in nuts and seeds, avocados, and fish (especially salmon), as well as in olive and canola oil. Eat fresh fish once a week and use olive oil freely in the diet, preferably uncooked in salad dressings and dips. Eat nuts and seeds regularly. Butter is healthy in moderation, and should always be used in place of hydrogenated fats such as margarine. Flaxseed oil (1 to 2 tablespoons daily) and evening primrose oil (1,500 to 2,000 mg daily) are also excellent supplemental sources of essential fatty acids. You can also boost the nutritional quality of your milk by taking a daily supplement of Neuromins by Martek. This is a fish-oil supplement high in DHA, a substance found to be markedly low in the standard American diet and particularly in breast milk.

Hydrogenated fats, especially margarine, and any products containing hydrogenated fats should be avoided as if your life depended on it. (It does!) The process of hydrogenation changes fats in such a way that they are chemically unrecognizable by the body. Their consumption has been associated with cardiovascular disease, elevated cholesterol levels, and even decreased immunity. They may also interfere with the baby's proper brain development, and the nursing mother should exclude them from her diet.

A WORD ABOUT DIETING

Whether or not you are breast-feeding, the postnatal period is a time when you should be replenishing yourself, not trying to diet. However, it is natural for you to want to shed those extra pregnancy pounds that are still hanging about on your hips, waist, buttocks, and thighs.

The safest and actually easiest way to do this is to establish a healthy diet that contains the maximum amount of nutrients with the minimum amount of unnecessary fats, empty carbohydrates (white flour, pastries, desserts, chips), and sugars. Don't count calories—instead, focus on learning to eat for nutrition and enjoyment, but not to fill emotional needs. Eat when you need to and how much you need to but not more. Avoid empty calories and go for nutrient-dense foods. Eat at home as much as possible; restaurant and fast-food meals are frequently laden with extra fat and calories. Keep snacks on hand such as vegetable sticks and a flavorful yogurt dip when you want to munch.

A safe weight-loss goal beginning 6 weeks after your baby is born is to lose 1 pound per week. Eating well, bypassing junk food, and adding moderate exercise to your lifestyle should help you achieve this goal without difficulty. Whatever you do, don't compromise your nutritional needs for a fantasy you have about the perfect body. If you imagine having a body without an ounce of fat or one wrinkle or sag, you're setting yourself up for a lifetime of disappointment. Strive for the healthiest body you can for your body type through eating well and getting moderate exercise. Add a positive outlook to this and you'll not only feel great, but you'll also glow with good health.

FOODS NURSING BABIES MIGHT NOT LIKE

Some breast-fed babies will tolerate just about anything Mom eats, even spicy foods, while other breast-fed babies are sensitive to even the smallest amount of certain foods, getting fussy or gassy within a few hours after you've eaten the offending food. If your baby has sensitive digestion, try to identify which foods upset her. The most common offending foods are spicy foods, caffeinated foods (especially coffee and chocolate), dairy products, peanuts and peanut butter, eggs, citrus fruits and orange juice, onions, wheat, broccoli, Brussels sprouts, raw cabbage, tomatoes and tomato sauce, corn, and soy products. Some babies are also upset by vitamin and mineral supplements (especially iron) taken by the mother.

The easiest way to identify the offending food is to experiment with your diet, eliminating all the foods from the above list and adding them back in one by one. If your baby gets fussy after one of these foods is consumed, eliminate ite for the first 6 months of breast feeding. Then you can reintroduce it to determine if it still upsets your baby once her digestive tract is more mature.

Some babies will have a fussy or "colicky" period each day regardless of whether or not you are consuming offending foods. Eliminating foods from your diet at your own nutritional expense is not healthy. If your baby is still fussing in spite of eliminating these likely offending foods, you might need to try another approach. Generally, babies outgrow fussy periods associated with colic by three months old. Speak with your pediatrician to be sure that there is not a more serious underlying problem. If your pediatrician tells you that your baby is fine and just has "colic," refer to my book *Naturally Healthy Babies and Children* for natural suggestions for treating colic and for keeping your own stress level down. A naturopathic doctor or herbalist specializing in pediatric care may be able to provide helpful suggestions and safe alternative therapies for your baby. An experienced mother may also have some tips for you. Please keep in mind that you must not compromise your own nutrition on a wild goose chase to identify offending foods. Your nutrition in the postnatal period is critical to your well-being, as well as that of your baby.

WATER, WATER EVERYWHERE

Although your body will produce milk even on only moderate fluid intake, drinking water abundantly throughout the day not only ensures plentiful milk production, but also prevents fatigue, depression, and constipation. Plan to drink ten 8-ounce glasses of water each day while you are breast-feeding. The easiest way to remember to hydrate yourself is by leaving glasses of water or water bottles where you spend the most time, such as in the diaper bag, next to your favorite chair, on your desk, or on the kitchen table or countertop. Also place a glass of water by your bed. Drinking water each time you nurse the baby and with each meal should provide you with plenty of liquid. Use your common sense but don't rely just on thirst. Thirst is not a reliable indicator of fluid needs, so push yourself to drink slightly more than you feel thirsty for.

Juice, soda, coffee, caffeinated tea, and other sweetened beverages are poor substitutes for water, as they contain lots of sugar (and calories!) and may actually cause you to excrete important nutrients such as calcium. Caffeine is a diuretic, which means you lose fluids. Water is the drink of choice for nursing moms.

HEALING AND HEALTHFUL RECIPES FOR NEW MOTHERS

Below are some of the foods I like to eat when I'm nursing my babies. They are high-energy, nutrient dense, and delicious!

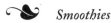 *Smoothies*

Smoothies provide an easy way to get a lot of nutrients at once. They're filling, too, and provide lasting energy. They are especially good when the weather is warm or when you need a quick meal but aren't very hungry.

> 1 cup organic vanilla yogurt
> $^1/_4$ cup organic milk
> 1 ripe banana
> $^1/_2$ cup fresh or frozen strawberries
> For increased nutrients (optional):
> 2 teaspoons flaxseed oil
> 1 tablespoon blackstrap molasses
> 1 tablespoon peanut or almond butter

Mix on high speed in the blender until the smoothie is nice and creamy. Enjoy as is, or blend in additional fruits such as fresh or frozen blueberries, peaches, and mango.

 Hummus

This popular Middle Eastern dip will keep for several days in the refrigerator.

> 2 cups canned or freshly cooked garbanzo beans (chickpeas)
> Juice of 1 lemon
> 2 tablespoons tahini (sesame seed paste)
> Garlic and salt, to taste

Mix on high speed in the blender or prepare in a food processor. Serve cool on pita bread, crackers, or as a dip for fresh raw vegetable sticks.

Tofu Dip

 1 pound firm tofu

 $^1/_4$ cup olive oil

 $^1/_4$ cup parsley

 2 tablespoons balsamic or apple cider vinegar

 1 tablespoon tamari (soy sauce)

 $^1/_2$ teaspoon dill

 $^1/_2$ teaspoon garlic powder

 $^1/_2$ teaspoon onion powder

 Salt (optional)

Blend until creamy. Will keep refrigerated for several days. Serve as for hummus.

RAW VEGGIES

Keep raw vegetable sticks in the refrigerator in a bowl of water. They'll stay fresh like this for several days and are an easy snack to grab for when you're hungry but unable to prepare a meal.

Serve with hummus, tofu dip, or any other healthy vegetable dip.

 Barley Stew

An excellent snack or part of a meal for early postpartum, barley stew encourages good milk production.

 2 carrots, diced

 2 celery stalks, diced

 1 large yellow onion, sliced thin

 1 parsnip, diced (optional)

 shiitake mushrooms, sliced (optional)

 2 tablespoons olive oil

 2 cups dried pearl barley

Sauté the carrots, celery, onion, and the optional parsnip and mushrooms in the olive oil until the onion is tender, 3–5 minutes. Transfer to a large pot and add the barley and 8 cups of water. Bring to a boil and simmer for 1 hour, or until barley is tender. Add salt to taste. Serve warm. This delicious stew will keep for 3 days in the refrigerator. Simply heat and enjoy!

Blueberry Muffins

You'll probably want to double the recipe, as these go fast!

> 1 cup unbleached white flour
> 1 cup whole wheat flour
> $1/2$ cup cane sugar
> 1 teaspoon baking soda
> 1 cup plain or vanilla yogurt
> $1/2$ cup canola oil
> 1 teaspoon vanilla (if you used plain yogurt)
> 1 egg
> 1 cup fresh or frozen blueberries

Preheat the oven to 350 degrees. Either butter a muffin tin or line it with paper muffin cups. In separate bowls, mix the wet and dry ingredients, then fold together. Fold in the blueberries. Spoon into muffin cups and bake for 30 minutes, until golden on top and cooked in the center. Cool on a baking rack. Makes 12 muffins.

 ### Complete Meal Salad

If you're attempting to eat light but want something filling and healthy, try this complete meal salad.

> 1/2 head romaine lettuce, broken up
> 1 carrot, grated
> 1 whole cucumber, peeled and sliced
> 1 cup garbanzo beans (canned is fine)
> 1/4 cup grated cheese
> 1/2 red pepper, thinly sliced
> 1/4 red onion, thinly sliced
> 2 tablespoons sunflower seeds (raw or dry-roasted)
> Olive oil and balsamic vinegar dressing, to taste

Toss well and enjoy!

Pasta Salad

This healthful and delicious salad will keep, refrigerated, for several days.

> 1 pound penne or rigatoni pasta, cooked until just tender
> 1 cup broccoli, slightly steamed

1 cup mixed beans (kidney beans and garbanzos are perfect)
$1/2$ cup sliced cherry tomatoes
$1/4$ cup cubed hard cheddar cheese
$1/4$ red onion, sliced
2 tablespoons chopped fresh basil
2 tablespoons olive oil
1 tablespoon balsamic vinegar
Salt and freshly ground black pepper (optional)

Chill slightly and enjoy warm or cool.

 Grandma's Chicken Soup
This is my grandma's recipe.

1 four-pound chicken
Carrots
Celery
Parsnips
Onion
Parsley
Salt and pepper to taste
Noodles (optional)

Buy a whole chicken (organic, though that's not my grandma's idea) and cut into quarters. Wash the chicken inside and out, then place it in a large pot with enough water to cover. Add generous amounts of carrots, celery, parsnips, and onion. Cook until the chicken is tender, skimming any foam that comes to the surface. Toward the end of the cooking, tie up a small bunch of parsley and put it into the pot ("the soup gets the flavor, but people don't all like parsley in their bowls," she says). The soup should cook for at least an hour and a half. Add salt and pepper to taste.

When done, remove the chicken and separate the meat from the bones. Place the meat into serving bowls and ladle the soup over the chicken, or serve the chicken separately. If desired, cook noodles and add to the soup.

Grandma said to be sure to use a lot of vegetables to make it taste sweet.

This can be made weekly, and leftovers can be eaten throughout the week as a complement to meals or as a snack.

Best Pumpkin Spice Cake

This is a filling and tasty snack, containing vitamin A–rich pumpkin and protein-rich walnuts.

> 2 cups whole wheat or unbleached white flour
> $1/2$ cup chopped walnuts
> 1 cup fresh or canned pumpkin puree
> $1/2$ cup milk
> 1 cup sugar
> 2 lightly beaten eggs
> 2 teaspoons baking powder
> $1/2$ teaspoon baking soda
> $1/4$ teaspoon salt
> 1 teaspoon cinnamon
> 1 teaspoon ground ginger
> $1/4$ teaspoon powdered cloves

Preheat oven to 350 degrees. Mix dry and wet ingredients in separate bowls, then combine. Pour batter into a greased and floured cake pan. Bake for 40 minutes or until top springs back when lightly touched. Cool in the pan for 10 minutes, then cool on a wire rack for 30 minutes.

 Sesame and Shiitake Mushroom Soup

> 1 teaspoon toasted sesame oil
> $1/2$ inch fresh gingerroot, peeled and cut into small pieces
> 1 carrot cut into julienne slices
> 4 ounces shiitake mushrooms
> 6 cups of vegetable or chicken broth
> 4 ounces soba or somen noodles
> 1 tablespoon tamari
> salt to taste
> 4 ounces tofu, optional
> 1 tablespoon fresh cilantro

Sauté the vegetables in oil, leaving out the cilantro. Cook 4 minutes and add broth. Stir into the noodles and add the tamari. If using tofu, add at this point. After 10 minutes turn off heat and add cilantro. Serve warm.

Asian Tofu Wrap
2 tablespoons sesame oil
1 pound firm tofu
2 cups washed and finely chopped kale
1 large, finely grated carrot
2 cloves garlic (optional)
2 tablespoons rice wine vinegar
2 tablespoons tamari
2 tablespoons fresh, chopped cilantro
4 12-inch whole wheat tortillas

Sauté tofu, greens, and carrots in oil until the tofu begins to brown and the vegetables become tender. Add fresh garlic, seasonings, and cilantro. Serve over warm tortillas.

Scallion and Ginger Chicken
1 tablespoon olive oil
2 boneless chicken breasts
1 tablespoon fresh, grated gingerroot
$1/4$ cup chopped scallion
2 cloves chopped garlic (optional)
$1/2$ cup vegetable or chicken broth
2 tablespoons rice wine vinegar
1 tablespoon tamari
1 teaspoon sugar

Brown the chicken on both sides in the olive oil, cooking 3–4 minutes per side. Cooking over low heat, add the ginger, scallion, and garlic, as well as the broth, rice wine vinegar, tamari, and sugar. Cook for 5 minutes longer. Serve warm with rice.

Oatmeal Raisin Cookies
1 cup raisins
$1/2$ cup water
2 cups rolled oats
2 cups unbleached white flour
1 teaspoon baking powder
$1/4$ teaspoon salt

$^1/_2$ cup canola or walnut oil

$^1/_2$ cup butter

1 cup sugar

2 eggs

2 teaspoons vanilla

1 cup chopped walnuts

Preheat oven to 350 degrees. Thoroughly combine all ingredients. Bake for 10–15 minutes or until golden brown. Cool on a wire rack for 15 minutes.

 ### Lentil Soup

Easy to prepare, makes great leftovers, and can be a meal, a complement to a meal, or even a hearty snack.

1 tablespoon olive oil

1 cup dried green lentils

1 bay leaf

1 medium yellow onion, diced

1 large carrot, diced

1 red bell pepper, diced

1 tablespoon fresh, chopped mint (optional)

$1^1/_2$ teaspoons salt

2 cloves crushed, fresh garlic (optional)

1 16-ounce can pureed tomatoes

black pepper to taste

Sauté the onion, carrots, and pepper in the olive oil, leaving out the mint. Add the lentils, tomatoes, bay leaf, and 6 cups of water. Bring to a boil, and then simmer for 1 hour, adding the mint about 5 minutes before finished cooking. The lentils should be soft when done. Add black pepper to taste if desired.

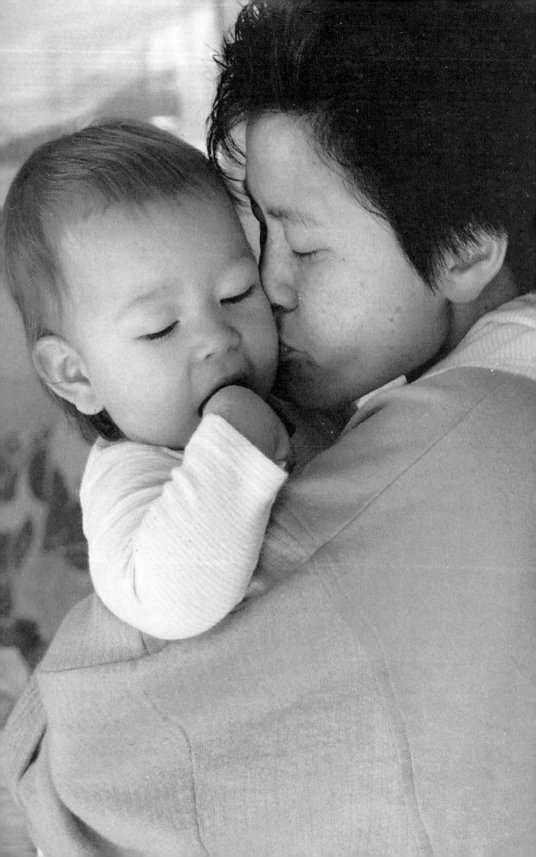

SEVEN

Into the First Year

Women today, trying to compose lives that will honor all their commitments and still express all their potential with a certain unitary grace, do not have an easy task.
Mary Catherine Bateson, *Composing a Life*

❧ WONDERING WHO YOU ARE ❧

The voices of mothers are clear to those who listen. Motherhood is an incredible joy and blessing. Our children enter our hearts and there they stay forever. Motherhood is also a demanding profession, one for which the rewards are of the heart, not the kind that pay the bills. And at moments, mothering feels like a thankless task—diapers, dishes, laundry, mopping, carpooling, and more dishes. Even mothers who have full-time household help and lives of luxury know there is no certainty in motherhood—life happens. Life happens to mothers, to children, to families. And through it all, we continue to love. Matters of the heart are sacred, but at the same time make us vulnerable. From this can come indomitable inner strength and grace.

In the midst of the daily business of motherhood, many women wake up to the feeling that they are made for more than dishes and diapers. Mothers are artists, dreamers, tennis players, doctors, teachers, engineers, nurses, writers, free spirits, academicians, and musicians. Some women become mothers before realizing they have other talents; others put their talents on hold for motherhood; still others navigate the waters of combining personal dreams with the fine art of mothering. In accepting the cloak of motherhood, do we necessarily need to forgo our identities as individual women? The answer to this is a complicated yes and no.

EMBRACING MOTHERHOOD AND ENJOYING YOUR BABY

When you become a mother, your priorities must necessarily shift so that baby comes first. For most women this shift happens so naturally that they know that if a ship were sinking, they'd save their children before giving a thought to anyone or anything else. Your baby is the apple of your eye. During the first couple of months after birth, women instinctively want to hold their babies, rocking them long after they are asleep at the breast or bottle.

Holding, talking to, carrying, and touching baby have now been well documented to improve the baby's rate of growth and provide optimal stimulation for neurological and cognitive development. Anthropologist Ashley Montague, in his brilliant book *Touching*, explains the importance of touch for physical, emotional, and mental health. In another of his books, *Growing Young*, Montague discusses the concept of exterogestation, the need for the human infant—one of the few mammals born totally dependent on their mother—to be treated as if in the womb for the first 8 months after birth: virtually continually held, kept with mother, and nourished from the mother's body through breast milk. Science is fast validating Montague's theories, with evidence that babies who are touched often grow healthier and stronger, and those who are breast-fed are cognitively and immunologically advanced.

In accepting motherhood, we must also accept that it is our responsibility to make our babies our priority—and for most, it is our love and delight to do so. Some mothers feel trapped by the full-time care babies require. This is sad and unfortunate, and too often a result of external pressures and anxieties faced by the mother, that prevent her from enjoying a time that can never be repeated or re-created later. As one mother said to me recently, "Work will always be there—my children will grow up."

This is all true, but mothers also need to nourish themselves as people. In truth, a healthy mother is more likely to raise a healthy child. Her own sense of fullness and satisfaction will spill over to her child. If full-time mothering provides all the satisfaction you need, you will be able to devote yourself to that path with little inner conflict. However, being home full time is not enough if you are frustrated and irritable. As children grow up they can sense resentment, and the last thing you'd want to do is become resentful of your child because you did not fulfill your own creative needs. Furthermore, I don't believe it's fair or healthy for women to build their entire lives around their children. Children also need to feel free to pursue their talents and dreams, with a healthy sense of balance between those with whom they have a relationship and their own path.

There is a natural progression that occurs in motherhood and our own development as women. It does seem that Mommy provides children with something special that is hard to get from a substitute, though some stay-at-home daddies do quite nicely. As children grow, they gain more independence, and we have increasingly more hours in the day on our hands to pursue our own passions. This does not mean that our passions must sit on a shelf until our kids go to college; but, rather, that we must creatively weave our patterns into this fabric of motherhood, which, as they grow, becomes easier to do.

This is healthy for children, too. They want to be the center of our world, but they don't always want us to be the center of theirs. Sometimes they just want us there on the sidelines for support. Ideally, we can patiently let our passions grow over time, so that our children blossom inspired by our example. Ideally, we have enough flexibility in our own work that we can pick and choose to be in the center of their lives whenever they need us to, and always quietly on the sidelines to give support.

⸙ "I FEEL LIKE I CAN'T GET ⸙ ANYTHING DONE"

During the first year or so after your baby is born, you'll probably hear yourself saying this or feeling this way at least a dozen times—sometimes a dozen times in one day. Simple things like washing a load of laundry get put off for days. Folding the clean laundry feels like a monumental accomplishment. The idea of pursuing your own passions seems hopeless and impossible. And during the first months after birth, indeed it may be hard to get much more done than read a book while you feed the baby—but chances are you'll doze off even trying to do that.

Taking care of a baby is a 24/7 occupation. To some extent, we just have to surrender to this for a while, gathering enough support to keep us sane. At first you may feel overwhelmed but don't mind because you recognize this is just part of having a newborn. But by about 3 months postpartum, you're probably starting to feel a bit caged in and a maybe a little bored by the routine (or lack of it!). You may not be sleeping much, and your beautiful baby is more demanding of interaction and attention. Most of the time you love this, but sometimes you need a break. Though you previously loved holding baby long after she fell asleep, now you yearn for that nap when you can put her down for 2 hours.

There are several things that will help you cope with this time when, in truth, it is hard to get much accomplished aside from the demands of baby care. First, although you're probably tired of reading this by now, it's essential to get adequate rest. Lack of rest makes even the most patient mother cranky and overwhelmed. You may want to get everything done while the baby is asleep, but you'll be better off napping when he naps and then trying to get things done when he is having a quiet alert time. Pick your priorities and set reasonable goals. If, for example, you like a clean house, don't try to clean it all at once, but instead spend 30 minutes a day picking up. One mother I know would wash her baby's face and wipe the baseboards with the cloth on the way to putting the wet cloth in the laundry room.

Just do a little at a time. Also, combine efforts. Make cleaning your workout, too, by putting on some good music and strapping baby to your back in a pack. Carrying the baby this way also frees you to do other things you love. It can be done if you like to cook, paint, sculpt, hike, garden, or any number of activities.

By 3 to 6 months postpartum, you may be ready for a little time away from your baby—perhaps just an hour or two to yourself, or alone with your mate. If you want to take time just for yourself, this is easy—just do it when your partner can watch the baby. If you are breast-feeding, nurse the baby well before you go. If you use a bottle, leave expressed milk. Even just 2 hours to sip tea and browse at a bookstore, or grab a movie or a meal with a girlfriend, can recharge you until the next opportunity arises.

Need a date with your partner? Similarly, go out for just a couple of hours, nursing baby well before you leave, or you can go for longer if you leave pumped milk. To care for baby, find someone you trust enough that you can relax while you're out. Pick a relative, close friend, or neighbor. Eventually, you can find a regular baby-sitter if you want one. It's normal to call home several times to check on the baby when you first go out. Our oldest is 16 and our youngest is 7 as I'm writing. My husband and I just started to go out regularly, and we always call home to check in at least once during the course of an evening. It really lets the kids know we care and reassures them that we're okay, too.

If you are a full-time mom and need some regular time to yourself during the work week, look for a college student who can come in for a couple of hours during the day, or a neighborhood middle school or high school student who can come in for a couple of hours a week after school. This is a fairly inexpensive way to get reliable help—teenage girls are generally great with babies. Take this opportunity for a bath, a walk, to catch up on correspondence, or to work on projects or passions.

By the time the baby is 6 to 8 months old, you'll still have days when you feel exhausted, but you won't get tired as easily as you did a few months earlier. You'll find yourself able to get some things done while baby naps or after he goes to sleep. Your life will always be fuller and more demanding than before you had children, but you'll have some breakthrough moments of finishing projects, being alone, or time to make dinner without having to stop to feed or comfort a crying baby. Also, as your baby learns to sit up on her own, new doors of opportunity open up for you. You can prop up baby with toys and pillows and do all manner of things. Your free time might be limited by the baby's attention span and appetite level, but you'll begin to feel more like yourself. By the time baby is a year old, you'll have some semblance of a routine, and will be much more comfortable with the art of multitasking.

♫— YOUR BODY —♫

It is important to recognize that both physical and emotional health problems are common after childbirth, although most women do not speak to their care providers about them (Brown and Lumley 1998). In fact, 94 percent of postpartum women in one survey reported tiredness, backache, sexual problems, hemorrhoids, perineal pain, depression, or a combination of these. Women who had operative births (cesarean, vacuum extractor, forceps) were even more likely to report these problems (Brown and Lumley 1998, Saurel-Cubizolles et al. 2000), as were women who experienced financial stress (Saurel-Cubizolles et al. 2000). Furthermore, in one study women felt they were poorly prepared for the amount of discomfort they would feel months after birth, even after uncomplicated birth experiences (Kline et al. 1998). Women deserve better preparation for birth and postpartum, better birth experiences, more postpartum support, and better recognition and understanding of, and support and treatment for, common postpartum complaints.

PERINEAL DISCOMFORT

By about 3 months after birth your body has probably made an almost complete recovery from birth—your uterus is back to its pre-pregnant size, your belly no longer looks 5 months pregnant, and your perineal tissue has healed.

However, if you had an episiotomy or a tear that was stitched, you may still have significant perineal discomfort. For most women, this occurs as periodic aching in the perineum, and for many women it interferes with their interest in sex. If you have persistent perineal pain, speak with your midwife or other care provider. You can also do gentle perineal massage with almond oil to which has been added vitamin E oil ($\frac{1}{2}$ ounce of vitamin E oil to $3\frac{1}{2}$ ounces of almond oil) and oil of rose geranium (10 drops). Gently work the perineal tissue with your fingers for 10 minutes daily to break up adhesions and soften the area. Your partner can also do this gently for you.

PELVIC-FLOOR WEAKNESS AND URINARY INCONTINENCE

Your pelvic tone may be a bit weaker than before birth, and you're more likely to dribble a bit of urine when you cough, sneeze, or jump. This just means you need to tone up your pelvic floor with pelvic-floor exercises (Kegels). A small number of women will experience a prolapse, or slipping down, of the organs in the pelvic cavity. Most commonly this happens to the uterus (uterine prolapse) or bladder (cystocele). Treatment of these conditions also requires pelvic-floor exercises, and generally takes more time and patience than does mild urinary incontinence. Pelvic-floor exercise must be done daily, usually 200 to 400 Kegels per day. It will take time for you to build up to this number, so start with 30 to 50 daily and increase by 20 to 50 per week. Just like any other muscles in your body, pelvic-floor muscles tire easily until tone is developed. Be persistent and tone will improve.

Women who experience uterine prolapse may first suspect something is wrong because they feel a lot of pressure or bulging in their vagina, or a sensation of having a tampon in when they aren't wearing one.

There are varying degrees of prolapse, from a mild first degree—where the cervix and uterus have slipped down slightly—to a fourth degree, in which the cervix protrudes from the vagina. Prolapse is not a medical emergency, but it can be uncomfortable and debilitating, particularly from the anxiety or threat that "everything will fall out." Limit your activities, as you have to avoid heavy lifting, jumping, and any other effort that puts strain on the uterine ligaments. Surgical repair of the prolapse is often the recommendation. The procedure involves tacking the uterus and bladder back up in the pelvic cavity. In extreme or persistent cases, hysterectomy may be recommended. This is rarely, if ever, necessary in women of childbearing age, and a uterine prolapse does not preclude giving birth vaginally to more children. Furthermore, with diligence, persistence, and proper pelvic-floor exercises, combined with pelvic tilts, pelvic organ prolapses can heal naturally.

CLASSIC CHINESE HERBAL FORMULA FOR UTERINE PROLAPSE

Herbs alone cannot fix a uterine prolapse. Treating a uterine prolapse requires time—as much as 1 to 2 years—during which you diligently repeat pelvic-floor exercises daily, follow good nutrition, avoid fatigue, and don't lift heavy objects. However, the following formula is considered the classic herbal preparation for treating prolapse.

TONIFY THE MIDDLE AND AUGMENT THE QI (BU ZHONG YI QI TANG)

12 grams astragalus

9 grams atractylodis

9 grams ginseng (or 18 grams codonopsis)

6 grams citrus peel

6 grams dang gui

3 grams bupleurum

3 grams cimicifuga

3 grams honey-fried licorice

Take daily as a tea or in the form of dried herbal powder capsules. (See Resources for Chinese herbs.)

EXERCISE

By 3 months you can begin to exercise regularly, and by 6 months postpartum you can generally resume a fairly active exercise program. Just be sensitive to your body's needs and responses and don't push yourself beyond your current limits. Avoid lifting heavy weights from a standing position for at least the first 6 months to prevent uterine prolapse.

YOUR BREASTS

By now breast feeding is much easier, and by 6 months your breasts will have mostly stopped leaking, though they probably still get engorged when full of milk. You'll notice that if you're away from the baby for several hours, you'll look forward to nursing just to relieve the fullness! You still run the risk of developing mastitis if you don't prevent engorgement or nurse when you are engorged, especially if you are run-down or undernourished. Take care to prevent this from happening. Again, adequate rest, good nutrition, and plenty of fluids are your best postpartum tools.

202 — Into the First Year

HAIR LOSS

Beginning around 5 months postpartum, many women report significant hair loss—their hair comes out in clumps in the shower and when they brush it, and they wake to find hair on their pillows. This can be frightening. It seems to be related primarily to hormonal changes that occur in the postpartum period, possibly to lower thyroid function during this time, and possibly to nutrient losses associated with pregnancy (and breast feeding). Keeping up your nutrition and taking a prenatal vitamin will prevent hair loss from nutritional causes. The problem usually resolves on its own, and the hair loss probably just amounts to loss of the increased hair thickness that was gained during pregnancy. If hair loss persists, becomes significant, or causes you anxiety, speak with your midwife or other care provider.

INCREASED SUSCEPTIBILITY TO COLDS AND INFECTIONS

Fatigue, anemia, stress, and similar factors can increase your susceptibility to colds and infections, especially after the first 6 months postpartum. Frequent colds are not only additionally exhausting to you, but they also prevent you from having energy for your baby. Paying attention to your own health needs during this time is essential for your wellness and that of your whole family. Don't let yourself get run-down, keep up your nutrition, and take time to relax in whatever ways bring you pleasure. Be careful not to rely on sugar, chocolate, sodas, or coffee to keep you going—this only further depletes your immunity.

MOTHER'S IMMUNE TONIC

This herbal tincture (see pages 242–44 for more about tinctures) is an excellent immune-supporting blend that also prevents exhaustion and recurrent illness. It is safe for nursing mothers.

1 ounce astragalus tincture
1 ounce elderberry and flower syrup
$1/2$ ounce ashwaganda tincture
$1/2$ ounce eleuthero tincture
$1/2$ ounce nettle tincture
$1/4$ ounce aniseed tincture
$1/4$ ounce licorice tincture

Mix the syrup and all of the tinctures together in a 4-ounce bottle.
Dose: 1 teaspoon, in warm water, 2 or 3 times daily. Continue for up to

6 months if needed. In addition, take echinacea tincture, 1 teaspoon twice daily, if you feel yourself getting sick.

BACKACHE

Women who have had an epidural commonly report backache, which may persist as long as a year postpartum. Pregnancy, particularly if posture was poor, as well as the strain breast-feeding positions can place on the back and neck, can also increase the likelihood of persistent backache. Gentle stretching exercises, warm baths, and regular massage will bring relief. If your backache is birth-related, and you feel bitter, disappointed, or resentful about your birth, expressing these feelings can also be helpful. The human being has a remarkable ability to somaticize emotions—that is, to store in the body our unexpressed feelings.

Herbal therapies can temporarily or permanently relieve musculoskeletal tension, and are a good companion therapy to those suggested above. Chamomile tea is an excellent musculoskeletal relaxant that is safe for breast-feeding mothers.

Aching Back Tincture
$^1/_2$ ounce cramp bark
$^1/_4$ ounce black cohosh
$^1/_4$ ounce motherwort

Combine these 3 tinctures in a 1-ounce bottle.
Dose: Take 1 teaspoon up to four times daily, either in plain water or added to chamomile tea

HEMORRHOIDS

To protect against hemorrhoids, pay attention to your diet and prevent constipation. A high-fiber diet with plenty of fresh fruits and vegetables and an adequate intake of water is your best bet. Straining during bowel movements aggravates hemorrhoids. To treat mild hemorrhoids see chapter 4. For natural therapies to treat persistent hemorrhoids, seek the help of a qualified herbalist or naturopathic physician.

The following preparations can be used while breastfeeding (see pages 242–44 to learn how to make a tincture):

Internal Tincture Therapy

1 ounce nettle tincture

$^1/_2$ ounce yellow dock tincture

$^1/_4$ ounce collinsonia tincture

$^1/_4$ ounce horse chestnut tincture

Combine these tinctures and take 1 teaspoon twice daily for 6 weeks.

 Topical Therapy

$^1/_2$ ounce witch hazel tincture

$^1/_2$ ounce lavender tincture

$^1/_2$ ounce plantain tincture

$^1/_2$ ounce white oak bark tincture

Combine the tinctures. Dilute 1 teaspoon of tincture in 1 tablespoon of water. Dab liquid onto the affected area with a cotton ball several times daily. Alternatively, soak a cosmetic pad in the dilute solution and apply to the hemorrhoid, leaving in placed tucked against the hemorrhoid. Repeat several times daily. Continue treatment for 2 weeks.

❧ MOTHERHOOD AND YOUR CAREER ☙

There is a theory that working mothers breed behavioural problems in their kids, that it is quantity time, not quality time, that counts. But I don't know one woman who doesn't need to work. So the working mother is damned if she does and damned if she doesn't—a famliar and frustrating situation.
Anita Roddick, *Business as Unusual*

By 3 months many women face the difficult decision of whether to return to work, and those who don't have the choice are preparing to go back. For some of you this might be a relief and something you look forward to with enthusiasm. For those of you who must return to a job but would rather be home with the baby, this can cause confusion and resentment. Most mothers spend a lot of time feeling guilty about decisions they make when these decisions require them to take time away from being with baby. This can be very painful and may cause chronic stress.

The issue of motherhood and career is a challenging one. A friend of mine was somewhat of a computer genius in college and throughout graduate school. Before having children she had a lucrative career and made more money than her husband. She continued to work throughout pregnancy and into her first year of motherhood, putting the child in daycare. Then she realized she wanted to be home with her growing family. Now, having taken off from her career for the past 17 years to raise her three children, she has lost her footing in the computer world, which has grown too fast and furiously for her to have retained a competitive edge. In returning to the work world, she has had to look to other employment avenues.

Many women realistically share concerns about their place in their own professions, and don't want to give up what they worked hard to gain. Many women also want to maintain a feeling of personal and financial independence—a practical consideration for mothers. One solution mothers find is to take a long maternity leave, then slowly pick up part-time hours or, whenever possible, bring work home. Other women find that giving up their professional life is a worthwhile trade for being home with growing children.

This is also a time to think very creatively about what kinds of options exist or opportunities you can create to work from home or to have your baby with you. Many more women are coming up with home businesses. If this is not an option, remember that you can continue to nurse your baby and have a close relationship in spite of less time together.

❧ TEETHING BABY, SLEEPLESS NIGHTS ❧

During the first few months, you're probably getting about half the sleep you really need. Chances are your partner needs more sleep, too. In some families, when Dad works full time and Mom stays home, the dad sleeps in another room while the baby is very young in order not to be a zombie at work. This can put an unfair strain on you if you're the one up with baby, and prevents the loving relationship and intimacy you share when sleeping together. If you are both having sleepless nights, be careful to take time to nurture and be gentle with each other. This will help prevent the bickering and short tempers that are common when sleep is lost.

Where your baby sleeps can have a big impact on how well you sleep. Some families find they sleep better when baby is in bed with them; others discover that despite their best intentions, they can't get any sleep with baby there. Many parents who wanted to have a family bed have reported to me over the years that their babies sleep better when put into their own bed. Some solve this by attaching an extender bed next to their own, moving the baby's crib into their room, or putting a mat or bed in their own room for the baby to sleep on.

When your baby reaches 5 to 8 months old, she will probably start teething. Some babies' teeth come in more easily than others. Most babies like to nurse more when their teeth start to come in, so breast-feeding babies will probably wake up during the night for a meal. Be tender with yourself. Allow yourself to return to taking naps with baby if you have the luxury to be home, and certainly try to catch up on sleep on the weekends. Herbal teas and remedies that promote relaxation and nourish the nervous system will do more for your energy level than coffee. You can also prepare Mother's Milk Tea Blend (see page 107), or give other safe, relaxing teas to baby to help calm him. Topically, you can rub small amounts of valerian tincture prepared in brandy onto the baby's gums. It smells strange but works wonders to ease teething pain. Clove oil is another possibility, but dilute it well, as it is caustic and can be irritating to sensitive gums.

⅔⌒ STILL NURSING ⌒⅔

Women who choose to nurse older babies often begin to receive pressure from family members, friends, and even the pediatrician to put the baby on solid foods or discontinue breast-feeding. Usually the pressure builds around the time the baby reaches 6 months old. Physically, there is no reason the baby cannot still receive primary nourishment from the breast. First babies are often quite content to nurse exclusively for most of the first year; subsequent children are likely to want solids earlier, as they want to be part of eating when everyone else eats.

Babies cannot easily digest starches and proteins before 6 to 8 months of age, so giving these sooner may do nothing more than bother their digestion or, at worst, lead to food allergies. When you start to feed solids, give pureed fruits and vegetables and gradually work up to grains and protein foods. Avoid dairy foods until the end of the first year, and then give only yogurt.

Emotionally, prolonged breast feeding through the first year is a wonderful gift to give to your baby. Internationally, the average age of weaning is 2 years old, and in some cultures children nurse up to 4 years. We have one friend, now in his mid-20s, who grew up in Ethiopia. The youngest of seven children, he was breast-fed until he was 7 years old. He can remember returning home from grade school to nurse!

Developing friendships with other mothers who choose to breast-feed beyond a year can bolster your confidence and provide the courage to stick to your convictions even in the face of family pressure. Your mother-in-law may give you cross looks or suggest you'll be more comfortable nursing your 1-year-old in another room at family gatherings. Try not to take it personally, and be prepared on how you will respond. You could set boundaries on nursing in public, you might decide to nurse your older child only at bedtime and naptime, or, as many women are now doing, you could nurse openly and freely and take a stand for the rights of mothers to breast-feed their babies as needed. If you do, you won't be alone!

Many mothers begin to get tired of breast-feeding toward the end of the first year. You may feel ready to have your body back to yourself. I remember when my fourth child finally weaned (at age 2½) what a delight it was to wear any kind of dress or shirt I wanted and not have to think, "Can I nurse in this?" I went for a long time refusing to wear dresses with buttons in the front! If you've nursed your baby for a whole year, you've given him an amazing start in life. Whether you continue after this is your choice. Breast milk after the first year is less nutritionally significant for children—it really comes down to emotional and immunologic nourishment, the foundation for which has already been laid but can always be built upon. At this point, do what is best for both you and the baby emotionally and physically.

Regardless, it is certainly a reasonable time for your child to eat more solids and rely less exclusively on breast milk for her calories and nutrients. If your baby still nurses at night and this is disturbing your ability to rest and function, it is also a reasonable time to get your partner to help wean baby from the nighttime nursing. This can be hard to do, and even painful if your baby cries a lot, but daddy can be there to rock and comfort his child as she learns to sleep through the night. Many breast-feeding families wait until baby is closer to 18 months to wean from night nursing, and some choose just to let it continue until the baby naturally sleeps easily through the night. This is a challenging decision. There certainly seems to be some element of habit associated with night feedings. Of course if the baby is feverish or sick, on-demand nursing is the best medicine. Make sure you eat exceptionally well and drink plenty of fluids as long as your baby is still breast-feeding.

❦ NEW-MOTHER MOODS ❧

In the first year after birth you'll go through many ups and downs. Your menstrual cycle is likely to return, but your hormones will continue to fluctuate. Stress, sleep loss, baby's changing needs, and needs of other family members will all play a role in how you feel. You'll have good and bad days, easy and hard nights. Though at times you won't believe it, all in all, things will get smoother and easier. Sometimes the baby will cry and you'll be at a loss for what to do, but mostly your baby will delight you with adorable smiles, precious looks, and positive feedback. When you have a hard day, remind yourself that you are still postpartum and this is all still new.

You're on a perpetual learning curve as a parent. Just as soon as you figure out what the kids like to eat for dinner, they're 16 and you have to figure out the ground rules for letting them drive in a car with other teenagers. I don't think the learning curve ever stops; it's just that we mellow with the job, gain a certain amount of trust in the fact that they grow up well in spite of us, and learn that love and attention go a long way. So be gentle with yourself. Nourish yourself. Cry freely when you need to. Slam a door if you are angry or frustrated (I've even broken a dish or two!), take a walk if you're going out of your mind, keep up with your physical wellness and appearance because this keeps you feeling good about yourself, and nurture deep friendships with other mothers.

❦ ISOLATION AND SOCIAL NETWORKS ❧

A few weeks ago I had a dinner at my home to which I invited two friends, each of whom has a young baby. I live an hour from them; they live 5 minutes from each other. They remarked that they never see each other regardless of their best intentions.

New mothers can get so wrapped up in everyday life that they forget to make time just to visit and chat. Yet it is this talk among women that keeps mothers healthy and prevents them from feeling alone and isolated. During the first few months after your baby is born, it is natural to stay focused on being home, but as baby gets to be 6 months, make it a priority to get together with other mothers. It is in honest conversation that we find our own sanity. We realize our trials and struggles are not unique, but instead are universal, and in this realization we feel not only healthy and normal, but also part of something bigger than ourselves and the world of diapers and sleepless nights. With this comes a sense of pride that can elevate the experience of motherhood to a new level of significance.

᎒ PROLONGED POSTPARTUM DEPRESSION ᎒

The best way to prevent postpartum depression is to take excellent care of yourself and maintain a strong support network well into your first postbirth year. Receiving help is one of the most significant factors in preventing postpartum depression. Although you can't control whether others give you help, you can control whether you ask for it. Postpartum depression is a serious problem and one that diminishes your ability to enjoy this special time with baby. Do what you can to prevent it, and ask for help if you suspect you have postpartum depression. The causes can be emotional, but they can also be hormonal. Physical health problems at 6 to 7 months postpartum, including back pain, tiredness, and urinary incontinence, are all associated with the development of postpartum depression. These are all treatable problems. Sexual problems, increased frequency of colds and coughs, bowel problems, and relationship difficulties are also contributing causes, and, like the other problems, can be resolved (Brown and Lumley 2000). Getting help can make a difference in the quality of your life.

For a complete discussion of postpartum depression see chapter 5, and refer to the discussion on this topic in Sally Placksin's book *Mothering the New Mother*. Contact a postpartum depression support group near you for help and resources in your area. Talking with other women who have been through postpartum depression and come out the other side will give you courage and confidence to face your own healing. Interestingly, one study shows that women who did not return to work before 6 months postpartum had a healthier mental status than did those who went back to work during this period (Gjerdingen et al. 1991).

᎒ PARENTING ISSUES ᎒

As your baby grows and begins to teeter into the world of toddlerhood, you and your partner will face new issues of parenting. Although some couples enter marriage and parenting with clear ideas and agreement on how to raise and guide, most figure things out along the way. Parenting and discipline values stem from many sources—the ways in which we liked or didn't like how our own parents raised us, subconscious patterns, social values, religious values, and positive role models we've had such as friends' parents and teachers. As your baby grows, he pushes boundaries—not deliberately, but naturally at first, and increasingly deliberately as time goes on. Regardless of how lovingly you parent, your child will present you with challenges. The idea is to be there to respond and to respond wisely and gently.

We also set patterns in our children by our own example from the very beginning. Furthermore, while we might choose to raise our children differently from the way our parents did, we can sometimes go too far in another direction. For example, adults who were raised in a strict environment and want to raise their own child more liberally might overcompensate and set too few boundaries, inadvertently creating a tyrant. As baby grows, read parenting books with your partner and talk about how you want to raise your child and how you expect to deal with a variety of issues (bedtime, picky eating, tantrums). Speak with other, more experienced parents to get tips and tricks. Stay open-minded to the moment.

Learning to parent together can be a joy if you keep your communications clear and continue to learn from each other and your child as you go along.

❧ RELATIONSHIPS, SEXUALITY, FERTILITY, ❧ AND BIRTH CONTROL

By 6 months postpartum, according to one study, about 89 percent of couples have resumed a sexual relationship. Of these, 83 percent of women reported sexual problems in the first 3 months after birth, declining to 64 percent by 6 months. Problems include painful intercourse, vaginal dryness, vaginal tightness, vaginal looseness, painful orgasm, bleeding or irritation after sex, and loss of sexual desire (Barrett et al. 2000). Many women are also afraid to conceive again so soon after birth, and therefore may be more hesitant to have intercourse. Some of these problems are resolved with time and only slowly and gently resuming your sexual intimacy, and, of course, choosing effective birth-control methods. If you have persistent problems in your sexual relationship, however, especially with either physical or emotional pain, speak with your midwife or a sensitive care provider.

Having a baby can bring a new dimension and new meaning to your own identity as a sexual being and to your sexual relationship with your partner. You see yourself as a mother now, as does your mate. For some couples, the experience of creating a life together and now bringing this life into being and raising him is deepening and profoundly bonding, enhancing the connection you both feel. For some men this is very arousing, but some men now see their wives as nonsexual mother figures, and this can be unsettling. You might be feeling less than in the mood for a sexual relationship after a full day of nursing, working, cooking, giving, and caring. The potential for tension in the postpartum sexual relationship is high; therefore, parents with a young baby need to keep communication open and loving. You may need to seek support if your sexual relationship is at an impasse. You might also be surprised at the intensity of your emotions surrounding the sacred parts of your body, which have recently opened wide to birth your baby, especially if the birth was difficult. This is normal. Find someone you trust and who has the experience and knowledge to help you sort out some solutions. Getting more physically comfortable, processing the birth, and finding other ways to deepen your intimacy are all part of the road to healing. Whatever you do, don't internalize the problem as your fault.

Fertility resumes anytime in the weeks or months after birth. Although ovulation is less likely to occur in nursing mothers in the first 6 months postpartum, breast-feeding is not a guaranteed method of birth control, and many unsuspecting mothers have conceived while breast-feeding and find themselves with two in diapers 10 months later. Remember, you ovulate 2 weeks before you menstruate, so you can get pregnant before you realized you were having a cycle again! To avoid a pregnancy too soon, choose an appropriate, safe, and effective method of birth control. At any time in the months after birth, begin to chart your cycle, cervical mucus, and basal body (resting) temperature, and combine the calendar and rhythm methods with condoms. Speak with your midwife or other care provider about what birth-control options are right for you at this time.

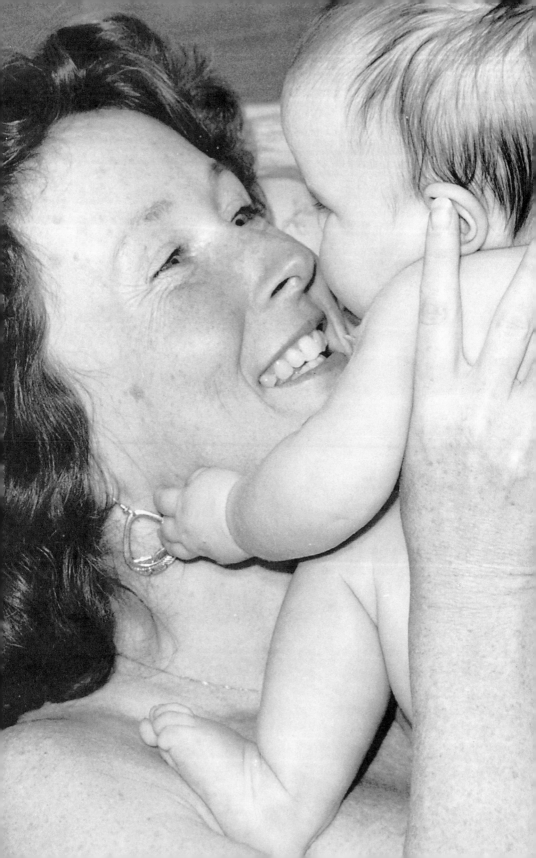

EIGHT

Replenishing Yourself: Body, Mind, and Spirit

*To put a child on Earth, an immense amount of creative
intelligence flowed from the Great Spirits, through nature
itself into your body, heart, and mind—remaining now, as an
integral part of your own spirit. This energy is yours forever.
Like a pocket, deep and filled with magic seeds of creativity
and healing, this is the source of unconditional loving from
which every wise woman since the beginning
of time has drawn her strength.*
Robin Lim, *After the Baby's Birth: A Woman's Way to Wellness*

his chapter is just for your pleasure. Your pleasure and peace are the
root, rock, and center of what you bring to your family. When you feel
rested and replenished, you glow from the core of your being, and this glow
spreads warmth and comfort to those around you. When you feel nourished,
you are better able to nourish those around you. When your cup is empty,
you have little to share; when your cup is full, it runs over to fill those around
you. Why nurture yourself? Jennifer Louden puts it well in her guide to
women's nurturing, *The Woman's Comfort Book:* "Because self-nurturing is
survival. Women take care of others every day. But how often do we turn our
wonderful nurturing ability toward ourselves? . . . When we nurture others
from a place of fullness, we feel renewed instead of taken advantage of.
And they feel renewed, too, instead of guilty. We have something precious
to give others when we have been comforting and caring for ourselves and
building up self-love." And as Rabbi Hillel once said, "You have a solemn
obligation to take care of yourself because you never know when the world
will need you."

❧ NEW-MOTHER MEDITATIONS ❧

Deena Metzger, in *Writing for Your Life*, reminds us of the power of retreat and withdrawal as a tool for self-renewal. "We withdraw," she says, "not only from the concerns of the world and its preoccupations but from the incessant monologue and concerns within ourselves, in order for something new to come into being." As a new mother, it is easy to have a running stream of inner thoughts telling you that you're not doing enough, not doing things as well as other mothers, not being a good enough mother, and a host of other negative messages. This can be mentally and emotionally exhausting, leaving you feeling you can never rest because there is always some more you must do or something you must do better. Mothers need to find ways to calm these inner voices and affirm for themselves what beautiful and dedicated mothers they are.

How do we calm these inner messages and replace them with healthier, more productive self-talk? It really comes down to practice—learning to deliberately catch yourself when you're giving yourself a hard time and replacing the thoughts with productive, affirming messages—sort of like reprogramming our inner computer. I prefer to think of it as nurturing our mind.

Affirmations are simple to do. Tell yourself what you want to think often enough and you create a self-fulfilling prophecy. Ask yourself what you might say to a best friend or child who was beating herself up emotionally—and say those things to yourself. Try these:

- I am worth nurturing.
- I deserve to nurture myself every day.
- I am a great mom.
- I have time in my life to do what I need to do.
- I deserve to do things at the pace of a new mother.
- My life is filled with joy and abundance.
- I am surrounding myself with people who love and support me.

Create your own messages based on what you need to affirm. There are many books filled with inspirational sayings and affirmations. Pick a few gems and write them on a piece of decorative paper. Tape them to the bathroom mirror, refrigerator, the corner of your computer, or all of these places as a reminder that you are all the things you want to be.

❧ NEW-MOTHER CHECKLIST ❧

When pregnant mothers first come into my practice, I give them a self-nurturing checklist. I tell them they can fill it out for their own information and keep their responses and score confidential, or they can show it to me and we can talk it over. The checklist has questions ranging from nutritional self-care to emotional self-care. Postpartum mothers can also give themselves a checklist of important things to do to remain well-nourished. Look over and answer these questions, checking off the items you're doing every day.

Based on your answers, are you allowing yourself to take care of *you?* Use these questions and your responses to inspire you to improve your self-nourishment. Then fill in the questionnaire. Answer in the spaces provided, on a separate piece of paper, or in a journal.

_____ I am eating well, paying attention to my current nutritional needs as a postpartum (breast-feeding) mother.

_____ I eat something fresh and natural every day.

_____ I allow myself to rest when I'm tired.

_____ I nap regularly or as often as I can.

_____ I drink enough fluids daily.

_____ I spend time in nature several times each week.

_____ I get enough sunlight most days of the week.

_____ I take good care of my physical health and get help for physical complaints.

_____ I take good care of my teeth.

_____ I get regular exercise.

_____ I make time to enjoy beauty (music, art, nature) in my life.

_____ I take time to relax and enjoy my life.

_____ I regularly do things that bring me joy and satisfaction.

_____ I ask for help when I need it.

_____ I forgive myself when I make a mistake.

_____ I take time to laugh.

_____ I make time for friendships and other important relationships.

**I COULD IMPROVE MY SELF-NOURISHMENT
IN THE FOLLOWING WAYS:**

1.

2.

3.

4.

5.

I COULD ASK FOR HELP OR SUPPORT TO DO THIS FROM:

1.

2.

3.

I DESERVE TO DO THIS BECAUSE:

1.

2.

3.

❧ CREATING TIME TO NURTURE YOURSELF ☙

You're a busy mom with a baby, possibly older kids, and maybe a career. How can you find time in your life to take care of yourself? This is a dilemma every mom faces, and indeed it seems like quite a challenge. But there are a few things you can do to create space for yourself without adding a 25th hour to the day and without cutting into your sleep time. Here is a list of creative tips for getting time to take care of yourself:

- Turn off the telephone for several hours each day or for one afternoon or evening a week. That's what answering machines are for. Schedule times when you answer the phone—and stick to that. It's amazing how much time and energy are frittered away in endless phone calls.

- Set specific times for housework, paying bills, returning calls, and other jobs that are constantly on your mind or in need of getting done. Focus on them during those times and accomplish all you can. Then put the task to rest. This will help you be more efficient in getting your work done, while also preventing you from being constantly haunted by jobs yet to do.

- Make a list of all the ways you "waste time" (e.g., getting stuck on the phone with someone who talks on and on, shopping in stores for things you could purchase by phone or computer, running errands each day rather than consolidating them) and brainstorm ways to be more efficient.

- Plan meals ahead for a week. Creating a weekly menu will really cut down on food preparation time, and make shopping more efficient because you know exactly what you need. If you plan well, you'll also have enough leftovers to almost eliminate lunch preparation. Thinking far ahead can also make your life easier—if, for example, you're making minestrone soup, double the recipe and put half in the freezer. For dinner a couple of weeks later, purchase a nice loaf of crusty French bread, slice some cheese, and heat your defrosted soup for an easy, delicious, and nutritious meal.

- Turn off the television and do something nurturing and fulfilling instead—make time for correspondence (letter writing is a fine art), read (or write!) a novel, plant a small garden, take a long bath, or do anything else that you'd enjoy.

- Hire a middle school or high school student to help you for 2 hours a week—or more—after school. This is an affordable way to get some time to yourself. Kids this age, especially girls, love caring for babies, so you're free to do things around the house that are nurturing for you, or to take care of business so you'll be able to relax later.

❦   YOUR PELVIC FLOOR   ❦

In Hindu the name for a woman's genitals is the *yoni*. It is considered a sacred word and is symbolized by an upside-down triangle. The medical word *vagina* means a "sheath," a term that arises from its association as a place for a sword, which both is male-centered and carries a violent connotation associated with cutting. Your yoni, having birthed your baby (if your baby was born vaginally), has gone through some dramatic changes in the past months, stretching large enough to allow the birth, possibly being cut or torn, and perhaps becoming tender for some weeks after birth. Many women who have had an episiotomy continue to experience perineal soreness for many months—even up to a year after birth. Furthermore, if you don't take care to exercise the muscles in the pelvic floor, you are more prone to pelvic-floor weakness, urinary incontinence, or organ prolapse after birth (see chapter 7).

Many women dissociate themselves from this amazing, sacred, and sensitive part of themselves, whether out of shame, childhood training, or embarrassment. Unfortunately, ignoring this part of our bodies can lead to lifelong health problems that worsen as we age. I strongly encourage women to love their bodies as part of their self-care practices, and to do pelvic floor exercises as a daily, or at least regular, part of their exercise routine. Pelvic-floor exercises incorporate tightening and lifting of the muscles that surround the vaginal area, urethra, anus, and perineum. Working up to 200 toning exercises in the course of a day as part of a general health maintenance program is ideal for long-term health, tone, pleasure, and the integrity of your amazing woman-body. When you tighten the pelvic-floor muscles, try to learn to do so without tightening your abdominal, thigh, or buttocks muscles at the same time. Really concentrate and focus on the yoni muscles and deep inside the pelvic floor. Visualize them tightening and toning as you work them. You can do pelvic toning exercises anytime—in the morning, before bed at night, when you are stopped at a red light or in traffic, before each meal (just smile—nobody will have a clue as to what you're doing!), while making telephone calls. You can also do them while having sex. You can learn to isolate these muscles while urinating—by stopping and starting the flow of your urine—but don't make it a habit to practice them while peeing, as this can lead to urinary stasis and increase your risk of urinary tract infection.

Pelvic-floor exercises are even more effective when incorporated into an exercise or yoga routine that includes pelvic tilts, pelvic lifts, and inversions such as shoulder- and headstands. If you are already experiencing some pelvic-floor weakness, don't despair. It may take several months to notice significant improvement in pelvic floor muscle tone, but if you stay committed to your exercises, you'll notice both improved tone in and better control of these muscles.

✄ FREE-MOVEMENT DANCE ✄

Work like you don't need the money, love like you've never been hurt, and dance like nobody's watching.

Proverb

Dancer, musician, and mother Gabrielle Roth takes the art of dance and free movement to a whole new level with her books, tapes, and dance programs geared toward moving with the emotions. She has her participants dance to music that emotes feelings of different elements and emotions—fire, water, and so on. The movements are uncontrolled and free but reflect the mood of the music. What Roth has done is create a program out of a possibility that's available to all of us in the privacy of our own homes, or in community centers or dance studios—allowing us to move our bodies freely and comfortably to express various aspects of our emotional lives and our connection to nature.

Dance is a highly therapeutic art form, and though many people judge whether they "can" or "can't" dance, movement is perhaps the most instinctive response we have—it's very hard to resist moving to music. Even babies in the womb do it. From the most primitive to the most technological societies, people make music and move to it. Maidens, pregnant women, new mothers, old women—all move their bodies to the music of their culture. We have a tremendous opportunity to use music therapeutically, as most of us have access to some form of stereo, CD, or tape deck, and there is abundance of musical genres available to anyone who can afford a few tapes or CDs.

Choose a few types of sounds you feel could inspire you to move your body freely (the privacy of your bedroom is just fine for dancing). Whether this is oldies rock 'n' roll or reggae, meditation music or Indian ragas, classi-cal music or hip hop—it's your choice. Do select music that lifts your spirits, brings you into deeper harmony with yourself, and inspires you, rather than music that's heavy or depressing. Let yourself move—even neck rolls and arm rolls are fine for a start. Don't judge yourself, but if you're comfortable doing so, use a mirror to see how you move. Look at where you could be looser, crisper, or achieve the movements that please your senses. Done regu-larly enough, you'll develop ease and comfort with free-movement dancing, and you'll increase your physical strength, stamina, and tone while relaxing your mind. As your baby grows, place him near you on a blanket and let him watch and enjoy the music. Eventually, as he becomes a toddler, he'll want to join in the fun. Children are incredible dancers—often very uninhibited in their movements—and great fun as dance partners.

✣ POSTNATAL YOGA ✤

Yoga means "yoke," or "union," and is about the joining of the body, mind, and spirit. Practiced during pregnancy, it can bring about great peace and foster the perfect blend of muscle tone and suppleness that often facilitates a smooth birth. Yoga is gentle enough to continue or even begin after the first 4 weeks postpartum, after the postnatal blood flow has ceased. There are many lovely yoga books from which you can draw more inspiration.

Below are several modified yoga *asanas,* or workout positions, that are specifically helpful for restoring tone to your body and proper placement of the pelvic organs, even as they encourage relaxation and mental peace and clarity. Gentle music accompanying your exercise routine enhances concen-tration and relaxation. Do your routine on a flat, firm, but comfortable sur-face such as a carpet, a yoga mat, or the grass outdoors. Remember to breathe deeply and peacefully with each position and movement, exhaling on the stretch and inhaling on the release.

POSTURE

As it was in pregnancy, excellent posture is essential for a healthy postpar-tum experience. In fact, backaches are one of the most common complaints women express in the first year postpartum. Neck, shoulder, and head pains, along with backaches, can all be prevented or reduced with excellent posture and proper alignment of the spine. The weight of your pregnant uterus may have encouraged you to allow your back to sway, and this must be corrected after the birth. Breast-feeding mothers and those who carry their babies in packs and slings have a tendency to slouch, and also get stiff in the areas mentioned.

Part of excellent posture is standing and sitting erectly, without swaying your lower back or slouching your shoulders. Bending properly (from the knees) and squatting, to lift objects—and to lift your baby and eventually your toddler—is also part of good posture. Careful lifting and bending can preserve the health of your back, whereas bending from the waist with straight legs to lift people and things puts tremendous strain on the lower back. How you carry your baby also has an impact on the health of your back. We tend to carry our babies on our hips, causing us to sway too far to the left or right. It is preferable to carry baby more to the front or the back to avoid lumbar strain. Similarly, proper support and a straight back while nursing, rather than a slouched back and slumped neck, prevents back and neck strain, and will preserve the long-term integrity of the back muscles and spine.

DEEP NECK RELAXATION (MODIFIED FISH POSTURE)

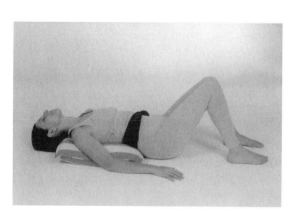

You can do this anytime in the postpartum, even hours after you give birth. You'll return to this position again and again as a nursing mother to work the kinks out of your neck and shoulders. Simply lie on your back on a firm surface with a pillow under your upper back, shoulders, and neck, but not under your head. Gently lower your head, effortlessly letting your neck stretch over the pillow, until your head is on the floor. Allow your shoulders to drop back and your arms to relax to the side. Remain in this position, eyes closed, for as long as you like.

A modified version is effective while you're sleeping: Lie in the same position, but instead of having the pillow under your upper back and shoulders, make a small roll of a soft pillow and place it under your neck. Let your head fall back. This will bring deep relaxation to your neck and shoulders.

TUMMY TONERS

New mamas are eager to get their bellies back into shape. These exercises are safe at 4 weeks postpartum, holding and repeating only briefly. Work up to more strengthening over the first several postpartum months. *Note:* Do not perform these tummy toners if you have had separated abdominal recti muscles without first speaking with your midwife or care provider.

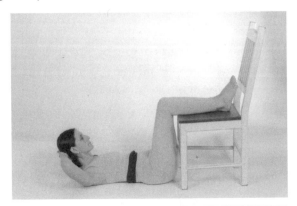

Form 1: Lie flat on your back with your feet on the seat of a chair and your knees bent at a 90-degree angle. Place your arms, bent, behind your head and pull in your belly button and tummy toward the floor. Gently lift your head and neck, keeping your shoulders mostly flat on the floor, and look toward your knees. Hold for 3 to 5 seconds, then repeat 5 to 20 times.

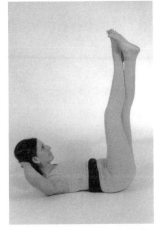

Form 2: Lie flat on your back with your legs raised almost, but not quite, perpendicular to the floor, feet crossed and knees slightly bent. From this position, repeat the head and neck lifts as in Form 1.

Form 3: This is more advanced, for after 8 weeks postpartum. Again, lying flat on your back, bend your knees so that your feet are on the floor near your buttocks. Place your hands behind your head as in Form 1. Now bring your left knee up and toward your chest while extending your right foot at a 45-degree and in front of you. At the same time, twist your right elbow toward your left knee. Hold for 3 seconds, then switch sides. Repeat 5 to 20 times on alternating sides.

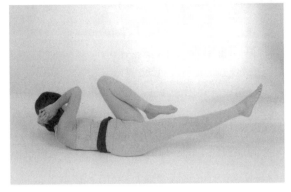

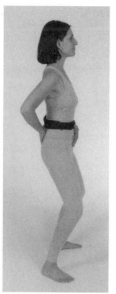
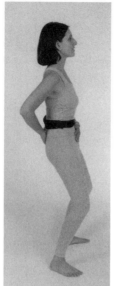

PELVIC TILTS

Stand with your feet shoulder width apart or slightly wider. Bend your knees so you are in a demi-plié (very partial squat). Tuck your pelvis far forward by arching the pubic bone toward the ceiling, then gently sweep your tailbone back toward the ceiling behind you. Repeat this rocking motion slowly and deeply (or more vigorously), to tone and strengthen the pelvic floor and the inner thighs.

GENTLE LEG STRETCHES

Sit upright with your legs as far apart as they can comfortably stretch with-

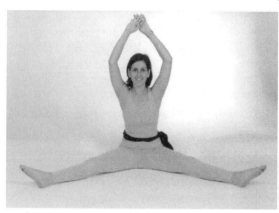

out causing you to slouch or feel pain. Raise your arms above your head, stretching upward from the waist, and lift up and out, leaning forward with your head going down toward between your feet. Hold for as long as is comfortable, using your inhale and exhale to deepen the stretch. Return to the center position and repeat 3 to 5 times.

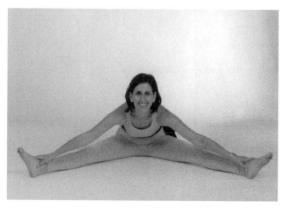

Now repeat as above, but stretch to the right and left, over first the right leg and then the left. Reach deeply with your breath, feeling the great stretching sensation in your waist, hips, and legs. This is fun to do with baby between your legs.

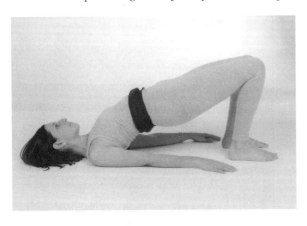

PELVIC LIFTS

Lying flat on your back, bend your knees and place your feet about 12 inches in front of your buttocks. Place your arms, straight at your sides, palms down, on the floor. Imagine a slender silver cord attached to your navel, pulling your belly up toward the ceiling or sky. Using your thigh and buttocks muscles, push your belly up toward the sky, keeping your back straight and firm. Hold for 5 to 20 seconds, return to the starting position with legs bent, and repeat 5 to 15 times. This tightens the belly, buttocks, thighs, and pelvic-floor muscles. (You can practice pelvic-floor exercises while your buttocks are in the raised position.)

⅋⸋ FABULOUS HEALING BATHS ⸎⅋

Baths are an underutilized, powerful tool for relaxing, and an inexpensive, respectable indulgence. All you need is a bathtub and you're most of the way there. What is especially lovely about bathing is that you can do it at home and at your convenience. Make a healing bath using herbal teas, essential oils, and bath salts, and select scents that soothe, relax, invigorate, and inspire. Healing baths will improve the quality of your sleep, relieve stress, reduce depression, soothe aching, sore muscles, and give you a quiet "time out."

TAKING AN HERBAL BATH

1. Choose a time when you can relax without interruption.
2. Play soothing music or create a quiet atmosphere.
3. Light candles in safe places around your bathroom.
4. Run your bath.
5. Have everything you need nearby—a towel, a robe or clothing for after the bath, a cup of water or tea, and your essential oil blend.

6. Add the bath oil, step into the bath, and relax for 30 to 45 minutes, adding more warm water to keep yourself comfortable.

7. After your bath, get into bed and rest, or allow yourself some time to continue to relax, making the most of your experience.

ESSENTIAL OIL BATH BLENDS

Essential oils are the distilled, extracted, and concentrated fragrances of flowers, gums, resins, and other plant components. Although many pure essential oils are expensive, you use such small amounts that they last a very long time. (I don't recommend synthetic oils and blends.) There are a number of companies that sell aromatherapy and essential oil products; see Resources for suggestions, and check at your local natural foods store. With the current popularity of aromatherapy products, there may even be a shop in your area that carries good-quality essential oils.

Instructions for Essential Oil Bath Blends

To prepare: Mix the recommended oils and store in a small glass or plastic bottle.

To use: Shake well and add 1 to 2 teaspoons of the oil blend to a warm bath. Stir the bathwater well to disperse the oil.

 Deep Peace Bath-Oil Blend

A pleasantly relaxing blend of scents to promote calm and improve sleep.

> 1 ounce almond oil
> 10 drops lavender essential oil
> 10 drops rose geranium oil

 Inspiration Bath-Oil Blend

Gently stimulating and invigorating to both mind and body.

> 1 ounce almond oil
> 10 drops lemongrass essential oil
> 5 drops orange essential oil
> 5 drops peppermint essential oil

Clarity Bath-Oil Blend

Improves mental clarity and function by gently stimulating mind and spirit.

> 1 ounce almond oil
> 10 drops rosemary essential oil
> 5 drops lime oil
> 5 drops peppermint essential oil

 Sensuality Bath-Oil Blend

Deeply scented, this blend is both deeply calming yet sensual.

> 1 ounce almond oil
> 10 drops amber essential oil
> 10 drops sandalwood essential oil
> 10 drops vanilla essential oil

BATH SALT BLENDS

Use bath salts in conjunction with or in place of essential oil blends.

Basic Bath Salt Blends

Bath salt blends comprise 1 cup of sea salt or mineral salts, $1/4$ cup of baking soda, and 50 drops of essential oil.

To prepare any of the blends described above as a bath, skipping the almond oil, use the essential oils for the therapeutic action you desire and add them to the basic bath salt blend. Try this blend:

 Sensuality Bath Salts

> 1 cup sea salt or mineral salts
> $1/4$ cup baking soda
> 25 drops sandalwood essential oil
> 15 drops amber essential oil
> 10 drops vanilla essential oil

Shake all ingredients well to prevent the oils from clumping. Place in a widemouthed glass or plastic bottle with a nice label, and store near the tub. Use 4 to 6 tablespoons of salts per bath.

Optional: To make your bath blend pretty, add 2 or 3 tablespoons of crushed dried flower petals or fragrant leaves to the mix. Lavender flowers, chamomile flowers, rose petals, rosemary leaves, mint leaves, blue malva flowers, and calendula flowers all make the blends look beautiful, and add their own scents to the mix as well.

BATH TEAS

Perhaps you've already tried the healing herbal blends for early postpartum and perineal healing. Prepare bath teas in a similar manner.

To prepare a bath tea: steep 2 large handfuls of your herbal blend in 2 quarts of boiling water for 30 minutes. Strain well, then discard the herbal material. Add the tea to your already drawn bathwater and relax.

Rosemary and Mint Blend
1 handful peppermint leaves
1 handful rosemary leaves

Flower Blossom Blend
1 handful lavender blossoms
$1/2$ handful chamomile blossoms
$1/2$ handful rose petals

ᘛ SHOWER SPA ᘚ

My favorite sacred place is the shower. Silly as it seems, it's the one place to which I can steal away nearly every day with no explanation necessary, usually at the start or the end of the day. It's perfect for relaxation. I turn on the water, sit down on the floor of the shower, and let the water run over me as I unwind. You can quickly transform a plain shower into an excellent spa with the addition of one of your essential oil blends, a loofah sponge, a soft towel, and an after-shower body splash. I like to treat myself occasionally to a bar of finely scented and nicely textured homemade soap, easy to find nowadays at most large natural food chains.

Place 1 teaspoon of essential oil blend on a washcloth and place this under the stream of water in the shower. The fragrance will rise through the shower and scent your bathroom. Then use the cloth to wash your body. Take your time to massage and be grateful for your body as you shower. You can even bring your toothbrush into the shower. Fresh body, clear mind, and clean teeth—you'll feel completely fresh when you emerge.

For a deeply relaxing shower—and a unique environment—light a candle in a safe place in the bathroom and take a shower in the near darkness!

After Shower Body Splash

Pour this splash into a mister body and spritz on after your shower, or splash it on if you don't have a spray bottle. Use this formula as a springboard to come up with your own fresh-scented and invigorating splashes, too. Mix together:

> 8 ounces distilled or plain water
>
> 4 ounces 80 proof vodka
>
> 20 drops lemon essential oil
>
> 20 drops rose geranium essential oil
>
> 10 drops peppermint essential oil

Shake well before each use.

SIMPLE PLEASURES FOR YOUR HAIR AND BODY

Right now is when a little treat like a special hair rinse or facial wash can be that something extra that makes you feel great—especially after a sleepless night with a teething baby. We all deserve to treat ourselves as the beautiful women we are—and women have known this throughout much of history. In fact, the use by women of body oils, hair perfumes, and cosmetics dates back to pre-biblical times. You can make many of these special preparations in your own kitchen. Use them either daily or whenever you need something special. And home beauty products are easy, affordable, and actually fun to prepare. Put your product in a special bottle with a nice label and a pretty ribbon, and this special gift can brighten up someone else's day, too.

HAIR CARE

When your hair feels nourished and healthy it can perk up your whole being. Make sure to take time to nourish yourself, head to toe!

Shiny-Hair Treatment

This oil nourishes the hair and scalp.

> 4 ounces olive oil
>
> $1/4$ ounce lavender essential oil
>
> $1/4$ ounce rosemary essential oil

Mix the oils and pour into a glass bottle. Comb a few drops into freshly washed hair or sprinkle a few drops onto your hairbrush and brush when your hair is dry. Or comb some into your hair just before you go to sleep. It's fine to use this treatment daily.

FACIAL STEAMS

Facial steams are as easy as making tea. In fact, they're basically the same as making tea. To make a facial steam:

1. Pick one or a selection of herbs from the box below.

2. Fill a 2-quart pot two thirds of the way with water.

3. Bring the water to a boil.

4. Add 1 large handful of your herbal blend and steep, covered, for 20 minutes.

5. While the herbs are steeping, clean your face well with soap and water or a cleansing scrub (see page 230).

6. Put a hot plate in the kitchen sink and place a large bath towel next to the sink.

7. Place the pot with herbs and water on the hot plate in the sink.

8. Cover your head with the towel, making a tent over the sink basin.

9. Keeping your head at least 18 inches above the pot, remove the lid and let the steam bathe your face. (Keep your head at a distance so that the steam is warm and penetrating but not burning.)

10. Breathe in the scents and steam, letting your skin be bathed and moistened.

11. Follow up with a cool herbal facial splash or spritzer (see below).

Caution: Do this very carefully. Steam can cause serious burns. Make sure your baby or toddler is safe in another room.

HERBS FOR FACIAL STEAMS

Burdock root	Mint
Calendula blossoms	Rose petals
Chamomile	Rosemary
Elder blossoms	Sage
Lavender	Thyme

Essential oils are a nice addition to a facial steam. Prepare as for an herbal steam, but when the water comes to a boil, turn it off, let cool for 10 minutes, then place the pot in the sink. Open the lid and add 5–7 drops of the essential oil(s) of your choice, then quickly close the lid. When your towel is in place, remove the lid and proceed as for the herbal steam.

CLEANSING SCRUBS

Facial cleansing scrubs are a gentle method of cleaning dead skin cells off your face and bringing increased circulation to your skin. They are generally made of ground grains and seeds, with herbs and essential oils added for healing and fragrance. Green clay is often added for its gentle drawing qualities that remove impurities from the skin, and it brings a nice consistency to the scrub. Below is an example of a simple cleansing scrub—get creative by using other seeds and grains, and by blending your own fragrances.

 Gentle Cleansing Scrub

Grind the following in a blender or food processor until they are a semi-fine, slightly gritty consistency:

> 1 cup rolled oats
> ¹/₂ cup almonds
> ¹/₄ cup lavender blossoms
> ¹/₄ cup rose petals

Add:

> ¹/₄ cup cornmeal
> ¹/₄ cup green or white cosmetic clay
> 10 drops rose or lavender essential oil

Shake all ingredients together and if warm or moist from the blender, let sit, uncovered, for 30 minutes. Store in an airtight container. Take out several days' worth at a time and keep near the bathroom sink. Keep the remainder in the refrigerator. To use, fill your palm with the blend, add enough water to form a paste, and spread over your face, gently scrubbing into your skin for several minutes. Rinse well with lukewarm water and follow with an herbal facial splash.

FACIAL SPLASH

Facial splashes, which turn into facial spritzes when you put them in a spray bottle or plant mister, gently tone the pores and are a great follow-up to facial steams and scrubs. They take minutes to prepare and will keep indefinitely. They'll also cool you down during a hot summer.

 Toning Facial Splash

> 4 ounces distilled water
> 2 ounces witch hazel extract (the regular kind from the pharmacy)
> 20 drops essential oil or oil blend of your choice

Store in a glass or plastic bottle and either splash or spray on, as desired. You can also apply with a cosmetic pad to clean oily pores. Rinse lightly with water after use to prevent dryness from the witch hazel. Shake well before each use.

 Vanilla Sandalwood Moisturizing Body Cream

This cream is very sensual and delightful—you'll love wearing it on your skin. It's also a nourishing hair oil: Brush a small amount into your hair before you go to sleep or before you go out into the sun to moisten and enrich dry hair.

> $1/2$ cup cocoa butter
> $1/2$ cup coconut oil
> $1/4$ cup almond oil
> 1 ounce beeswax
> 1 ounce vegetable glycerin
> $1/4$ cup water
> 1 teaspoon sandalwood essential oil
> 1 teaspoon vanilla essential oil

In a small pot, carefully melt the cocoa butter, coconut oil, almond oil, and beeswax. Allow to cool to room temperature, but do not allow the mixture to become solid. Place in a blender with the vegetable glycerin and water. Blend until well whipped and creamy. Turn off the blender and stir in the essential oils, mixing well. Add more essential oil, as needed, to achieve the depth of scent you desire. Pour into a clean, dry jar, and cap when thoroughly cooled. Store in a cool place. If water rises to the top, simply pour it off. This will happen only initially, as some of the water may separate from the oil.

Scent alternative: equal amounts of rose geranium and lavender oil.

BREAST MASSAGE

A nursing mother's breasts take a lot of wear and tear—and all women's breasts deserve a nourishing touch. Gentle breast massage is relaxing, and can also promote good circulation and lymph system drainage.

ᴄ᷍ *Breast Massage Oil*

If you include the poke root oil, use the following massage oil only topically on unbroken skin. Thoroughly wash the oil off your nipples before you nurse.

> 2 ounces poke root oil* (or 2 ounces olive oil, almond oil, or grapeseed oil)
> 10 to 15 drops rose geranium oil
> 10 to 15 drops sandalwood oil
> 5 to 10 drops tangerine oil

Massage your breasts in the same circular pattern that is used for a breast exam. Be gentle so you don't bruise your breast tissue.

*Specialty herb supply companies usually stock poke root oil (see Resources).

CREATING A HOME SPA

Showers, baths, and splashes are great for when you have only 10 minutes to an hour to do something special for yourself. But every now and then—even if it's only once a month or even once every couple of months—you'll feel energized if you have a half day to yourself, several uninterrupted hours, to really treat yourself to a spa day. This is something you can do at home, and doesn't require much more of an investment than the simple treatments you've already put together, some time, and the willingness to nurture yourself. A home spa day can incorporate simple body treatments, but is even more fulfilling if you incorporate some elements of body movement and creative expression.

Here's a sample home spa day:

10 A.M.:	30 minutes of dancing or yoga—enough to break a moderate sweat. Put on soothing music and allow yourself to relax deeply into your movements.
10:30 A.M.:	Drink water with lemon and read a chapter of an inspirational book.
11 A.M.:	Herbal shower, facial scrub, after-shower splash

11:30 A.M.:   Lunch (prepare in advance, or put on music and enjoy preparing) large salad with chicken or garbanzo beans, cheese and sunflower seeds; whole-wheat roll; minestrone soup

12:30 P.M.:   Creative journaling (see page 235) or pick up your book again. Put on soothing music while you read or write.

1–3 P.M.:   Take a walk or a short nap—perhaps curling up with that great book.

❧ QUIET TIME ALONE ❧

Quiet time alone nourishes the soul and allows us to return to the core of who we are. Solitude is a health requisite for busy mothers, whether this be 20 minutes at the start, in the middle, or at the end of the day; a formal weekly "retreat" time; or an evening alone every few weeks. How do you know when you need a quiet time? When noise makes you distressed, when you find yourself snapping at your kids to be quiet, when you hear your kids' voices still asking questions after they've gone to sleep, when you're irritated at the loud way your husband chews, when you can't even listen to music because you so badly crave the sound of silence.

It is nice to have a mix of time alone at home and somewhere away—at a park or in a library, for example. Time alone at home allows you to relax into your own self with minimal distraction—especially if you're clear about turning off the phone and not getting lost in the "should do's" of the household. You can put on cozy clothes and the soothing music of your choice— or have no sounds at all, if you prefer. Lie on your back in a comfortable location, close your eyes, place a cool flaxseed or herbal pillow over your eyes. Drink in the sensory quiet. Bathe in the stillness and emptiness of the moment.

If it's too difficult to accomplish complete relaxation at home, a peaceful time alone out of the house may be just the remedy. Choose a quiet place where you won't be bombarded by noise, stimulation, and distraction. A dimly lit café with soft chairs, tea, and a place to read a book or write in your journal is ideal. Visit a museum, botanical gardens, or a hidden corner of the local library. Take yourself on a cheap but therapeutic date for a couple of hours and come home refreshed, ready again to drink in the beautiful music of your family.

TIME IN NATURE

Nature is our truest healer and medicine when we are out of sorts, out of balance, and out of harmony. Being in nature quiets our inner noise, calms our breathing, and brings our heartbeat into a slower, more natural rhythm. Nature brings perspective, as we realize we are but a minute fraction of the universe, reminding us, too, that we are part of something bigger and infinitely wiser than ourselves. Our problems tend to decrease in intensity, as well.

For those of you already blessed to live in a natural environment, the best spa is right outside your door. A walk in the fresh air will improve sleep, mood, circulation, and muscle tone. City dwellers, find parks in your area that are safe for long strolls, either alone or with your mate or a friend, or with a canine companion, or with baby in tow in a pack. Look for places not too far a drive from home that offer natural beauty, space for contemplation and solitude, and room to walk and explore. Waterfalls clear the mind, open expanses really provide perspective and make for great stargazing, and long trails offer myriad opportunities to discover the small but infinitely beautiful miracles in nature—leaf skeletons, wildflowers, unfolding ferns, spiderwebs, and other intricate masterpieces. Marvel at it all and give thanks for your place in this great life.

❧ EXPLORING YOUR CREATIVITY ❧

Creative expression is one of my favorite forms of release: painting, singing, creating crazy sculptures for my garden out of old wine bottles and paint. After just a few hours of letting my spirit sing, I feel remarkably refreshed. It's also fun to watch my kids get inspired and begin to make things after I've been in a creative mode. Although you will have limited time while your babies are small to indulge in these passions and pursuits, keep a special box of supplies and magical items that you find and dream of turning into "art." Sometimes just keeping a dream box like this growing for a future project can be full of fun and mystery. Someday you'll have the time and inspiration to put it all together.

Similarly, if you have an artistic nature, or have had a professional life as an artist, don't let taking care of baby force your creative passions to die. Keep these alive even in small ways. Make time for your music, writing, or other creative passions. You deserve to surround yourself with beauty and magic, and this will serve as a lifelong inspiration to your family. By setting the example of being creative, inspired, and fulfilled people ourselves, we set the tone for our children also to be creative, inspired, and fulfilled.

〜 KEEPING A JOURNAL 〜

A journal is a sacred and private place to express your feelings, record the precious or painful moments of your day, jot down the wonderful things your baby did (or older children did or said), make note of great quotes you read, glue fortunes from fortune cookies, paste a special photo, dream, complain, doodle, vent, play. This journal can be something just for yourself, but it can also become a powerful legacy for the future. I recently had the privilege of leading a blessing ceremony for a pregnant mother. At this ceremony, one of the participants read an excerpt from her now deceased mother's pregnancy journal. The pages she read were written at the same stage of pregnancy that our mutual friend was in, and was a moving testament to a mother's love and expectations as she awaited the imminent birth of her child. We all cried as we were honored to hear these heartfelt words. This reinforced for me how special a treasure a journal can be. Don't let the notion of future generations reading your journal censor your words—you'll leave a legacy of what it's like to be profoundly human women and mothers.

There are so many beautiful books to choose from, and most are quite affordable—within $15 for a book that will last for at least 6 months even if you write every day—an amazing feat for any busy mother. Blank pages enable you to doodle, sketch, or otherwise embellish the journal. Lined pages are easier for neat writing, but I prefer plain pages and paste all kinds of remembrances, cards, sayings, small pieces of the kids' art, and love notes from my children and mate onto them. Sometimes I vent and then tear out pages. Other times I vent and then write an explanation so nobody ever thinks those feelings are permanent or personal about them. I refrain from venting much about my kids, but my poor husband has had some choice pages written about him over the past 17 years of my journaling through marriage!

There are also many books available with ideas for creative journaling if you want to get past the dear-diary style. You'll learn to write about your feelings productively, express yourself creatively, and explore your inner world through written expression. This can be an incredible journey through the labyrinth of yourself, as well as inexpensive and effective therapy!

Choose a journal that reflects who you are visually. When you pick up your journal it should bring you a sense of beauty and magic. If you can't find a journal you like, create your own with a blank art book from a craft store, some glue, clear acrylic glaze, and a postcard that you especially like. Glue the card onto the cover; paint this with the glaze, going over the edges of the picture onto the book cover to hold the edges in place and give it some shine; and allow to dry. It's that simple. Letting the family know that your journal is sacred to you will generally ensure adequate privacy. Or keep your journal in a special place that's all your own.

⅊ BE GENTLE WITH YOURSELF: EMBRACE ⅌ AND ENJOY YOUR BABY

As mothers, we are our own harshest critics—expecting nothing short of perfection for ourselves as we take into our care these seemingly perfect beings, our babies. We want to help our children preserve their perfection, and not impose on them our own foibles. We fret over every decision, wanting desperately to do exactly the right thing.

Alas, sometimes we bumble, stumble in the dark, make a less-than-perfect choice, lose our tempers, forget our adoration, and act horribly human. Occasionally we act like a mother cat, batting at her kittens when she is ready to wean. When we shoo away our kids, we cry and hope we have not harmed our perfect child for life. Sometimes we don't look at the perfect painting they made because we were talking on the phone to the plumber. Maybe we miss our 4-year-old's perfect pirouette because baby needed to nurse. But we hope they know how much we love them.

Motherhood is raw and pure. It is fierce and gentle. It is up and down. It is magic and madness. Single days last forever and years fly by. Toys are everywhere and then one day they are discarded. It is so easy to get twisted into knots over the many details of motherhood that we lose sight of the process for the goals, the journey for the destination. But motherhood—and childhood—is all about the journey. And while individual days and hours may last forever, and some nights seem endless, all too soon the journey is over and we wonder how we ever got there so fast. Be gentle with yourself as you travel, dear mother. Don't miss the scenery. Don't miss the conversation with your traveling companions. Laugh at the bumps and say "Ooh, aah" on the hairpin turns. Buckle your seat belt. You're a mom!

Gentle mother, may you walk in Beauty.

> *For each of us as women, there is a deep place within; where*
> *hidden and growing our true spirit rises. . . . Within these deep*
> *places, each one holds an incredible reserve of creativity and*
> *power, of unexamined and unrecorded emotion and feeling.*
> *The woman's place of power within each of us is neither white*
> *nor surface; it is dark, it is ancient, it is deep.*
>
> **Audre Lorde,** author of *Sister Outsider*

APPENDIX 1

Herbal Preparations

The instructions below show you how to prepare most of the medicinal remedies in this book. Although making all of your own medicines may be more than you want to do with a small child in arms, the preparation of teas, baths, and other simple remedies is easy. It's not too difficult to whip up a batch of baby bottom lotion or nursing mother nipple salve.

Enjoy and be well!

❧ PURCHASING HERBS ☙

If you are buying dried herbs in loose, bulk form from a health food store, a mail-order catalog, or another source, look for organic, non-endangered wildcrafted plants or at least organically cultivated plants. Preparations such as capsules and tinctures likewise should be prepared from organically grown herbs. Many herbs on the market have been fumigated with fungicides and insecticides during storage, and some are even irradiated. Check your sources.

All herbs and herbal products should have a fresh smell and the colors should resemble the color of the original plant material. Herb freshness will affect the potency and therefore the effectiveness of your treatments. A moldy odor indicates the herbs are not fresh. Look closely for insects, as one infested batch of herbs can let loose tons of bugs into your home. These will then infest other herbs in your pantry, and get into your foods as well.

❧ HERBAL PREPARATION ☙

It's quite magical to watch different herbs turn water, alcohol, and oils into lovely shades of gold, red, orange, green, and brown. Preparing your own remedies always seems to add a special magic to the medicines.

Common household supplies are all that's necessary to make everything from teas to salves in your kitchen. You'll need:

- A variety of glass jars, with lids
- Glass or stainless-steel pots
- Sharp knife
- Small funnel
- Mesh strainer
- Vegetable grater
- Measuring spoons
- Cutting board
- Vegetable oil
- Vodka
- Beeswax

There are some preparations you'll have to buy. These include essential oils, which require special equipment for extracting; and herbs that must be powdered, as it takes a special grinder to powder herbs to a fine enough consistency.

If you plan to use your own preparations as your primary medicines, look through this book and plan ahead. Tinctures, for example, take weeks to prepare; you'll want these on hand, as you don't have weeks to wait if you need a tincture today. Otherwise, purchase the herbs and preparations as the need for them arises. Most herbal preparations such as oils and tinctures will keep for up to a few years (refrigerate oils so they'll last); if you prepare small batches of medicines at a time, you'll find that little gets wasted.

༅ FORMS OF PREPARATION ༄

There are many possibilities for extracting the elements from plants needed for an herbal remedy. Different types of preparations are required for different situations. Water, alcohol, and oil are the most common bases (*menstruum* is another word for a base or solvent). Vinegar is also used by some herbalists, but as it is not suitable for all herbs, I reserve it for steeping fresh culinary herbs.

WATER BASES

Water is what most of our body is made of, as is the earth and as are plants. Our bodies accept water-based solutions easily. These include teas, infusions, decoctions, and syrups. Infusions and decoctions are also used for baths, washes, and compresses.

Tea is the most basic herbal preparation. To make a tea, steep 1 teaspoon to 1 tablespoon of a dried herb in 1 cup of boiling water for up to 20 minutes. Herbs with a high volatile oil content are easily extracted this way and should be covered during steeping to prevent loss of these oils. Catnip, chamomile, fresh ginger, lavender, lemon balm, peppermint, and seeds such as anise and fennel are in this category.

An infusion is a medicinal-strength tea. More herb material is steeped for longer in slightly more water. The result is a darker, stronger-tasting brew that is more potent than a beverage. Make infusions in 1-pint and 1-quart canning (mason) jars.

To make an infusion: In either a pint jar or a quart jar filled with boiling water, steep 2 ounces of chopped, fresh herb (1 ounce of chopped, dried herb) for $^{1}/_{2}$ hour to 8 hours. The amount of water in relation to plant material depends on the strength desired. The length of steeping time corresponds to the strength of the remedy and also on the part of the plant being used. Here are some general recommendations:

Roots: 1 ounce dried root to 1 pint boiling water; steep for 8 hours.

Bark: Prepare as for roots.

Leaves: Delicate leaves and those rich in essential oils are generally prepared 2 ounces fresh leaves (1 ounce dried leaves) to 1 quart water; steeped 1–2 hours. Steep thick leaves (such as uva ursi) up to 6 hours. When preparing leaves for nutritional purposes (such as nettles), steep up to 8 hours.

Flowers: Use 1 ounce dried flowers in 1 quart boiling water; steep for a maximum of 1 hour.

Seeds: Gently crush the seeds with a mortar and pestle, then steep for up to $^{1}/_{2}$ hour. The usual ratio is $^{1}/_{4}$ to $^{1}/_{2}$ ounce crushed seeds per pint of water.

Generally, dosage of an infusion ranges from $^{1}/_{4}$ cup to 1 cup, 2 to 4 times daily. Sometimes an infusion is sipped throughout the day.

A decoction is a concentrated infusion. This makes for a strong brew that enables you to take the medicine in smaller doses. It is an excellent way to take herbs that are difficult to tolerate in large amounts due to their strong taste. This method is especially suited to prepare nutrient roots such as dandelion and yellow dock because you can get concentrated doses of minerals without having to drink cupfuls of beverage. Leaves, flowers, and seeds are rarely decocted, as their constituents can be damaged by boiling.

To prepare, steep your infusion for up to 8 hours. Strain the liquid into a saucepan (discard the used plant material) and gently simmer until it is reduced to one half to one quarter of the original amount. Take care not to boil away all of the liquid. It takes approximately an hour to reduce a pint of liquid by half (down to a cup). Pour into a glass jar, let cool to room temperature, then refrigerate.

Unsweetened decoctions last in the refrigerator for up to 3 days. Two tablespoons of honey per $1/2$ cup liquid or about 2 tablespooons brandy per cup of liquid will extend the life of a decoction up to 3 months under refrigeration.

Dosage is usually 1 teaspoon to 1 tablespoon, 2 to 4 times daily.

A syrup is simple to prepare once you have made your decoction. There are two main advantages of using a syrup over a decoction. First, it's easier to take a small amount of a sweet-flavored medicine than any amount of an unpalatable one. Second, the large amount of sweetener in the syrup preserves the preparation, which helps it keep in the refrigerator longer than even a sweetened decoction. Simply sweeten the decoction by adding an equal amount (by weight) of sweetener. One cup of a decoction is 8 ounces, so a decoction of this amount requires 8 ounces of sweetener. I use $1/4$ to $1/2$ cup of honey per cup of liquid and find this adequate; honey is considered to be twice as sweet as sugar. Add the sweetener to the hot decoction; bring to the boiling point, stirring; then immediately pour into clean jars. Cool to room temperature, label, and refrigerate. Dosage is similar to a decoction but varies from herb to herb.

Taking an herbal bath is a rejuvenating ritual that's useful for all sorts of complaints: sore muscles, injured skin, exhaustion, irritability, congestion, and fever, to name a few. Be very careful to avoid burns from overly hot water.

A *footbath* is used to soak feet and is done in a basin of water wide enough for the feet and deep enough to reach at least above the ankles. Prepare by adding 1 quart of herbal infusion to enough hot water to fill the basin.

A *sitz bath* requires a quart of decoction, or a couple of quarts of infusion, placed in a shallow tub with enough water to reach hip level.

A *full bath* can be made two ways. One is to fill a cotton cloth or sock with at least 1 ounce of herbs, then fasten the closed cloth to the faucet and let the bathwater run through the sock while filling the tub. Squeeze the sock now and then to wring out the "tea." This makes a mild but pleasant herb bath. With the second method, prepare a couple of quarts of herbal infusion or decoction and then strain these into your tub of water.

If you keep the door to the bathroom closed, the aroma of the herbs will fill the air, as will any volatile oils. This adds to the relaxing effect of the bath. Herb baths are a nourishing gift to yourself during pregnancy. Floating herb flowers directly in the tub makes for a fun bath, but use a screen of some sort to keep the plant material from clogging the drain. Do not take baths if your waters have ruptured.

Poultices and compresses are ways of applying herbs externally to specific areas of the body. You can make a poultice quickly by mashing, bruising, or even chewing fresh herbs into a pulpy mass and applying as is to the affected area. You can also take fresh or dried herbs (moisten dried herbs with warm water first), mash them, and spread the mix on a thin cotton cloth, which you then apply. Place a hot-water bottle over the herbs or cloth to retain the warmth. Use a poultice for stings, bites, localized infections, wounds, boils, abscesses, swellings, and tumors.

To make a compress, soak a cloth in a hot infusion or decoction, wring out the excess liquid, and apply the cloth to the needy area. Replace the compress when it cools. As with a poultice, a hot-water bottle placed over the preparation retains heat.

A wash is just what it sounds like: You wash the area with an infusion or decoction. This can be done as an eyewash, for example, in treating conjunctivitis, or as a wash over a skin infection such as ringworm. It is an effective and simple external remedy.

ALCOHOL BASES

Alcohol is used for making tinctures. The amount of alcohol ingested when taking tinctures is fairly insignificant. If you are concerned about this, though, simply evaporate the alcohol by adding the dose of tincture to $1/4$ cup of hot water and let sit exposed to the air for a few minutes. You can now purchase many tinctures in a glycerin base, which, in addition to containing no alcohol, lends a slightly sweet taste. Alcohol is a valuable menstruum because certain plant substances can be extracted only by alcohol. The best alcohol to use is 100 proof vodka, which is 50 percent alcohol and 50 percent water. Grain alcohol (almost 200 proof) and brandy are other mediums. Brandy is nice in tinctures that will be used for very young kids because it's sweet, mildly warming, and lacks a sharp alcohol taste.

Tinctures are concentrated alcohol extracts of herbs. They are concentrated, quick-acting, have a shelf life of many years, and are convenient because you can transport them easily in small bottles. Because they are so concentrated, you need only a few drops, making them particularly convenient for those who can't prepare infusions or decoctions every day. *Note:* Do not use a tincture when the nutritional aspects of herbs are sought. For this, use a tea, infusion, decoction, or syrup.

Making tinctures at home is fun and much less expensive than buying them. Tinctures created with fresh plant material are superior to those made from dried herbs. Whenever possible, obtain fresh herbs for your tinctures or purchase tinctures made from fresh herbs. Place about 2 ounces of plant material in a pint jar. If you have gathered the herbs yourself, clean them by picking out damaged parts and brushing dirt off roots. Do not wash aboveground plant parts. Chop the roots, stems, and bark. Now fill the jar to the top with alcohol. This lessens the possibility of spoilage in the airspace between the tincture and the lid. Cap the jar tightly and label it with the name of the herb, alcohol content, and date. Store where it won't be exposed to direct sunlight, and give it a gentle shake every few days. If you see the liquid level going down, top it off with some more alcohol.

Some folks let their tinctures "work" for only 2 weeks. I prefer to let mine tincture for 6 weeks, starting at the new moon and ending at the full moon 6 weeks later. The moon affects the growth of plants, and it is wise to honor her as we make our medicines from them.

After 6 weeks, strain the alcohol tincture thoroughly from the plant material. This usually requires some vigorous wringing of the herbs in cheesecloth or cotton muslin to extract as much of the liquid as possible. Pour the tincture into well-labeled glass jars or tincture bottles (it is not necessary for the jars to be filled to the top, as it is in preparing the tincture) and store in a cool, dark place such as a pantry or the refrigerator.

The dosage of a tincture depends on the herbs used, the condition being treated, and the person's age and weight. Usually between 5 and 25 drops are taken 4 times a day. Store tinctures out of reach of children—an overdose could make them sick. Tinctures remain good for 2 or 3 years.

Liniments are tinctures that are prepared for external use in the treatment of muscle and ligament trauma. They tend to contain herbs that act as local stimulants (angelica, calendula, cayenne, cinnamon, wintergreen, for example) in order to bring deep warmth to the area and disperse blood congestion to reduce bruising. The alcohol (use vodka or other 100 proof alcohol) makes them quick absorbing and penetrating.

Prepare as for tinctures, or add essential oils to an alcohol base. Apply by rubbing enough into the skin to cover the area that is sore or bruised. Do not use on broken skin.

OIL BASES

Oil-based preparations you can make at home are herbal oils, salves, and ointments. Essential oils are highly concentrated plant extracts. They cannot easily be made at home and are rarely used internally, as their strength can be lethal. I have occasionally suggested the use of essential oils in this book as an external remedy, and caution you to store them in your home out of the reach of children.

Herbal oils, sometimes called medicated oils, are vegetable oils in which herbs have been infused. This is different from an essential oil, which is derived by extracting large volumes of concentrated, active chemical ingredients from plants. Herbal oils are used in the treatment of sore muscles, sprains, aches, infections, and irritated skin, and for massage. Many herbal oils mentioned in this book can be used on broken skin; however, do not use arnica oil.

To make an herbal oil, fill a clean, dry jar with dried herbs. Now fill the jar to the brim with oil. Almond, olive, and sesame oils are the most commonly used, but any vegetable oil is fine. Store at room temperature in partial sunlight for 1 to 4 weeks. Some herbs, such as garlic and rosemary, will keep well in oil for the longer time span; other herbs, particularly the more delicate plants and plant parts such as chickweed and rose petals, begin to spoil after 1 week. Additionally, hot weather causes the plants and oil to spoil more quickly, whereas plants extracted in a cool environment will keep longer before you must decant them. Avoid direct light and heat.

Infuse and store on a surface that will not be damaged by any oil seepage that may occur. At the end of the given time period, strain well and store in a cool, dark place or refrigerate. Oils will keep up to a year and sometimes more, and are considered good as long as the oil has not turned rancid. A rancid oil has a peculiar smell that is distinctly different from the smell of either the fresh oil or the plant being steeped. If you suspect the oil has turned, discard it and begin anew.

Salves are used to heal skin injuries: wounds, burns, stings, rashes, sores, and the like. There are several methods of making salves, all of which are effective. This first method is preferable because it requires the least cooking of the herbs and oil, and thereby retains more of the herbs' subtle properties.

Prepare an herbal oil using your salve ingredients. Then pour the herbal oil into a small pot. To this add grated beeswax, 1 tablespoon per ounce of oil. Heat over a low flame until the wax is melted. To test for readiness, put a small amount onto a teaspoon and place in the refrigerator. After a minute it will harden to its finished consistency. Salve should be firm and solid without being so hard that it can't be melted into your skin. If the consistency is correct, then pour the salve into small jars, cool to room temperature, cover, and store. If the salve is too soft, add more beeswax; if it's too hard, add more oil.

A second method is to place about 1 ounce of herbs and $1/3$ cup of oil in a small pot. Simmer, covered, for 2 hours on a *very low* flame. Add a bit of oil if necessary, and watch carefully to avoid scorching. Strain the herbs well through a cotton cloth or cheesecloth, squeezing as much of the oil as possible out of the plant material. Let the oil cool before you do this. Clean the pot and dry it (discarding the used plant material), then pour the oil back in, adding 2 tablespoons of grated beeswax. Melt this over a low flame, stirring constantly. Check for readiness as in the first method, then bottle and store.

A final method requires less watching. Mix 4 ounces of oil, 1 ounce of herb, and $1/2$ ounce of beeswax in an ovenproof pot with a cover. Bake at 250 degrees for about 3 hours. Strain through cheesecloth, bottle, and store.

Salves will keep for a couple of years if refrigerated and for about a year if unrefrigerated. To extend the life of your salve to the full 2 years, add 1 teaspoon of vitamin E oil or 1–2 tablespoons of an herbal tincture per 4 ounces of salve (while still warm, before bottling). Any herbal tincture will work, as it's the alcohol that helps it to keep. However, to increase the healing qualities of the salve, use a tincture with either skin-healing or antimicrobial properties. Echinacea and calendula tinctures both make a good choice for use in herbal salves.

Ointments are prepared exactly as are salves, but less beeswax is used in order to obtain a softer product. Cutting the amount of beeswax by half should yield a desirable consistency.

When you experiment in your kitchen pharmacy, above all enjoy yourself. Of course it's best not to be wasteful, but don't worry if you make a mistake and have to discard something. Compost piles love your mistakes! Try to be patient and learn from what works and what doesn't—the rewards are worth it!

Resources

Catalogs and brochures are available from most of the companies in this resource guide. Write or call for further information.

LifeCycles Midwifery and Herbal Wellness Center
Aviva Romm, CPM, Herbalist AHG
1931 Gaddis Road
Canton, GA 30115
770-751-7548
This is my practice and family business through which I offer a full line of herbal products for women and children, herbal and midwifery consultations in person and by telephone, and teaching engagements. We can also help you locate resources and supplies mentioned in this book.

SUPPORT AND RESOURCE ORGANIZATIONS

A.L.A.C.E. (Association of Labor Assistants and Childbirth Educators)
P.O. Box 382724
Cambridge, MA 02238
617-441-2500

American Academy of Naturopathic Physicians
8201 Greensboro Drive, Suite 300
McClean, VA 22102
703-610-9037
www.naturopathic.org

American Association of Oriental Medicine
433 Front Street
Catasanqua, PA 18032
888-500-7999

American Herbalists Guild
1931 Gaddis Road
Canton, GA 30115
770-751-6021
www.americanherbalist.com
If you are looking for a clinical herbalist in your area, this is the organization to contact. It also offers education materials, national conferences, and a journal for those seriously interested in studying herbal medicine.

Boston Women's Health Book Collective
240A Elm Street
Somerville, MA 02144
617-625-0271
This organization is an excellent resource for information on a wide variety of women's health issues and illnesses, provides well-written educational packets, and produced the important book *Our Bodies, Ourselves.*

Citizens for Midwifery
P.O. Box 82227
Athens, GA 30608-2227
316-267-7236
e-mail: SHodgesMWy@aol.com
www.cfmidwifery.org
This organization serves as the national clearinghouse for midwifery consumer support groups and acts as a consumer education group, educating the public about the advantages of midwifery care.

Depression After Delivery
91 East Somerset Street
Raritan, NJ 08869
Information request line:
800-944-4PPD
www.behavenet.com/dadinc
Education, information, and referral services for women with postpartum depression, with free information for individuals

and professionals, as well as those interested in volunteering to set up PPD support groups. Membership includes a newsletter.

Doulas of North America
13513 North Grove Drive
Alpine, UT 84004
801-756-7331
www.dona.org
This organization offers training in the postpartum support of new mothers.

I.C.A.N. (International Cesarean Awareness Network)
April Kubachka
1304 Kingsdale Avenue
Redondo Beach, CA 90278
310-542-6400 • Fax: 310-542-5368

International Childbirth Education Association
P.O. Box 20048
Minneapolis, MN 55420
612-854-8660
Excellent book catalog on pregnancy, birth, and related topics. Also a resource center for this information.

La Leche League International
9616 Minneapolis Avenue
Franklin Park, IL 60131
708-455-7730
800-La-Leche
www.laleche.org
An international organization with numerous locally placed League Leaders, women trained to support and educate women who want to breast-feed. Ardent supporters of breast feeding and the mother-child relationship.

Menstrual Health Foundation
104 Petaluma Avenue
Sebastopol, CA 95472
707-302-2744
Dedicated to empowering women during the years from menarche through menopause. Provides products and publications for menstrual health.

Midwives Alliance of North America
4805 Lawrenceville Highway
Suite 116-279
Lilburn, GA 30047
info@mana.org
This is a national midwifery organization dedicated to women's freedom and reproductive health, with members all over the globe. A good contact if you are trying to find or become a midwife.

National Association of Postpartum Care Services
800-45-DOULA
www.napcs.org
Resource for postpartum-care services with a national referral line.

Postpartum Support, International
805-967-7636
www.postpartum.net
National organization dedicated to helping women with postpartum depression. Offers a national counselor referral line.

United Plant Savers
P.O. Box 98
East Barre, VT 05649
802-496-7053
www.plantsavers.org

EDUCATIONAL RESOURCES AND MAGAZINES

Compleat Mother
Box 209
Minot, ND 58702
701-852-2822
"The magazine of pregnancy, birth, and breastfeeding." Very honest and uncompromising.

The Doula Magazine
P.O. Box 71, Dept. MT
Santa Cruz, CA 95063
Includes articles on pregnancy, birth, parenting, natural health care, toddlers, and more. "Always a nurturing read."

HerbalGram
P.O. Box 210660
Austin, TX 78720
An excellent and informative magazine that keeps abreast of scientific studies in phytotherapy.

Midwifery Today
P.O. Box 2672
Eugene, OR 97402
503-344-1422
A magazine for midwives and others involved with pregnancy and birth. Many pregnant women find this very informative as well.

Mothering **Magazine**
P.O. Box 1690
Santa Fe, NM 87504
800-984-8116
Perhaps the oldest of the alternative parenting magazines in the United States. *Mothering* seeks to honor and celebrate pregnancy, birth, parenthood, and children, and offers a wide variety of articles on these topics.

Sage Mountain
P.O. Box 420
East Barre, VT 05649
802-479-9825
www.sagemountain.com
Rosemary Gladstar Slick, founder of the California School of Herbal Studies, is a pioneer herbalist and the author of numerous booklets on herbs for women, men, and children. She offers a correspondence course in herbal studies.

Wise Woman Center
Susun S. Weed
P.O. Box 64-M
Woodstock, NY 12498
The author of *Healing Wise, Herbal for the Childbearing Year,* and *Menopausal Years* offers workshops and apprenticeships at her home, and travels internationally for speaking engagements.

BOOKS, HERBAL PRODUCTS, AND MOTHERING SUPPLIES

Avena Botanicals
20 Mill Street
Rockland, ME 04841
207-594-0694
Deb Soule grows, wildcrafts, and makes her own medicinal preparations from herbs especially for women. The mail-order catalog offers more than 150 tinctures.

Blessed Herbs
109 Barre Plains Road
Oakham, MA 01068
800-489-4372
A complete selection of bulk herbs, tinctures, and capsules, from a family-oriented, home-based business.

Bushy Mountain Bee Company
800-BEESWAX
Not an herb supplier, but a great source of pure beeswax for making salves.

Cascade Health Care Products
141 Commercial Street NE
Salem, OR 97301
800-443-9942
Offers a complete line of health products for pregnant women and midwives as well as many for babies and kids; good source for moxabustion supplies. Its *Birth and Life Catalog* (Imprints) offers a comprehensive book selection including numerous titles on prenatal health, pregnancy, midwifery, and a number of herb books, and its *Moonflower* catalog offers herbs, nutritional supplements, and homeopathic remedies.

Frontier Cooperative Herbs
Box 299
Norway, IA 52318
800-669-3275
Bulk herbs and health and beauty products at wholesale prices.

Glad Rags
800-799-GLAD (4523)
Washable cotton menstrual pads.

Herb Pharm
P.O. Box 116
Williams, OR 97544
800-348-4372
The highest-quality tinctures available from a company that takes extaordinary pride in its products, and also values its customers. The best echinacea around, among other things.

Herbalist and Alchemist
P.O. Box 553
Broadway, NJ 08808
908-689-9092
Also the highest-quality products made with great care to preserve the integrity of the plant. David Winston, the owner and formulator, puts together brilliant combinations.

Lunar Phases Calendar
Snake and Snake Productions
511 Scott King Road
Durham, NC 27713
Susan Baylies produces these annual calendars, which I've used for more than 15 years to record my menstrual and fertility cycles. They are the clearest and easiest calendars to use, and are very inexpensive.

Maine Seaweed Company
P.O. Box 57
Steuben, ME 04680
207-546-2875
Excellent sea vegetables harvested with complete respect for the health of the ocean.

Medela
800-TELL-YOU
Breast pumps and other equipment for breast-feeding mothers and babies.

Motherwear
320 Riverside Drive
Florence, MA 01062
800-633-0303
Well-made, chic casual and professional clothing for the breast-feeding mom.

Mountain Rose Herbs
P.O. Box 2000
Redway, CA 95560
800-879-3337
Beautiful catalog of bulk herbs, jars and tins, books, and premade formulas. Also very nice products for use in women's rituals such as candles, oils, and special art objects that are woman-affirming.

NF Formulas, Inc.
9755 Commerce Circle, C-5
Wilsonville, OR 97070-9602
503-682-9755
Prenatal and lactation vitamins.

Rainbow Light Nutritional Supplements
207 McPherson Street
Santa Cruz, CA 95060
800-635-1233
Prenatal and lactation vitamins.

Sage Mountain
P.O. Box 420
East Barre, VT 05649
802-479-9825
www.sagemountain.com
Offers herb products formulated by Rosemary Gladstar Slick, a highly experienced herbalist. I wholeheartedly recommend all of Rosemary's products as well as her book *Herbal Healing for Women*.

Bibliography

Abou-Saleh, MT et al. "Hormonal aspects of postpartum depression." *Psychoneuroendocrinology.* (1998 July); 23 (5): 465–75.

Acheson, LS and SC Danner. "Postpartum care and breast-feeding." *Primary Care.* (1993 September); 729–47.

Adinma, JI. "Sexual activity during and after pregnancy." *Adv Contracept.* (1996 March); 12 (1): 53–61.

Angier, Natalie. "Mother's milk found to be potent cocktail of hormones." *The New York Times.* Thursday, May 24, 1994. B5.

Akre, J. "Breastfeeding: pledging allegiance to ourselves." *Archives of Pediatrics.* (2000 May); 7(5): 549–53.

Arms, S. *Immaculate Deception II: A Fresh Look at Childbirth.* Berkeley: Celestial Arts, 1994.

Arvigo, Rosita. *Sastun: My Apprenticeship with a Maya Healer.* San Francisco: HarperCollins, 1995.

Astbury, J et al. "Birth events, birth experiences and social differences in postnatal depression." *Australian Journal of Public Health.* (1994 June); 18 (2): 176–84.

Baker, JP. *Prenatal Yoga and Natural Birth.* Berkeley: North Atlantic Books, 1986.

Baldwin, Rahima. *Special Delivery.* Berkeley, CA: Celestial Arts, 1986.

———. *You Are Your Child's First Teacher.* Berkeley: Celestial Arts, 1989.

Ball, Jean. *Reactions to Motherhood: The Role of Postnatal Care.* Cambridge, England: Cambridge University Press.

Barrett, G et al. "Women's sexuality after childbirth: a pilot study." *Archives of Sexual Behavior.* (1999 April); 28 (2): 179–91.

Belenky, M et al. *Women's Ways of Knowing.* HarperCollins, 1986.

Bensky, D and R Barolett. *Chinese Herbal Medicine: Formulas and Strategies.* Seattle: Eastland Press, 1990.

Bernazzani, O et al. "Psychosocial predictors of depressive symptomology level in postpartum women." *Journal of Affective Disorders.* (1997 October); 46 (1): 39–49.

Bernt, KM and MA Walker. "Human milk as a carrier of biochemical messages." *Acta Pediatrica Suppl,* (1999 August); 88 (430): 27–41.

Berggren-Clive, K. "Out of the darkness and into the light: women's experience with depression after childbirth." *Canadian Journal of Community Mental Health.* (1998 Spring); 17 (1): 103–20.

Bick, DE and C MacArthur. "Attendance, content and relevance of the six week postnatal examination." *Midwifery* (1995 June); 11 (2): 69–73.

Bing, E and L Colman. *Laughter and Tears: The Emotional Life of New Mothers.* New York: Henry Holt, 1997.

Blumenthal et al. *The Complete German Commission E Monographs Therapeutic Guide to Herbal Medicines.* Austin: American Botanical Council, 1998.

Bove, M. *An Encyclopedia of Natural Healing for Children and Infants.* New Canaan, CT: Keats, 1996.

Brown, S and J Lumley. "Physical health problems after childbirth and maternal depression at six to seven months postpartum." *British Journal of Obstetrics and Gynecology.* (2000 October); 107 (10): 1194–201.

———. "Maternal health after childbirth: results of an Australian population based survey." *British Journal of Obstetrics and Gynecology.* (1998 February); 105 (2): 156–61.

Buchart, WA et al. "Listening to women: focus group discussions of what women want from postnatal care." *Curationis.* (1999 December); 22 (4): 3–8.

Caplan, C. "Postpartum realities." *Mothering.* 1989 Spring: 73–76.

Chan, SM et al. "Special postpartum dietary practices of Hong Kong Chinese women." *European Journal of Clinical Nutrition.* (2000 October); 54 (10): 797–802

Cohen, N. *Open Season: A Survival Guide for Natural Childbirth and VBAC in the '90s.* New York: Bergin and Garvey, 1991.

Crawford, A. *Herbal Remedies for Women.* Rocklin, CA: Prima, 1997.

Cummings, AG and FM Thompson. "Postnatal changes in mucosal immune response: a physiological perspective of breast feeding and weaning." *Immunol Cell Biol,* (1997 October); 75 (5): 419–29.

Dai, D and WA Walker. "Protective nutrients and bacterial colonization in the immature human gut," *Advanced Pediatrics,* 1999; 46: 353–82.

Dankner, R et al. "Cultural elements of postpartum depression." *Journal of Reproductive Medicine.* (2000 February); 45 (2): 97–104.

Dash, B. *Embryology and Maternity in Ayurveda.* New Delhi: Delhi Diary, 1975.

Davis, E. *Women's Intuition.* Berkeley: Celestial Arts, 1989.

Davis, MK. "Review of the evidence for an association between infant feeding and childhood cancer." *International Journal of Cancer Supplement,* 1998; 11: 29–33.

Duerbeck, NB. "Breast-feeding: what you should know so you can talk to your patients," *Compr Ther,* (1998 June–July); 24 (6-7): 310–8.

Dunham, C and The Body Shop Team. *Mamatoto: A Celebration of Birth.* New York: Penguin, 1992.

Edwards, D et al. "A pilot study of postnatal depression following cesarean section using two retrospective self-rating instruments." *Journal of Psychosomatic Research* 38, 111–17.

Elliot, SA and JP Watson. "Sex during pregnancy and the first postnatal year." *Journal of Psychosomatic Research.* 1985; 29 (5): 541–8.

Ellis, DJ and RJ Hewat. "Mothers' postpartum perceptions of spousal relationships." *Journal of Obstetric Gynecologic Neonatal Nursing* (1985 March–April); 14 (2): 140–6.

PL Engle, et al. "Child development: vulnerability and resilience," *Soc Sci Med*, (1996 September); 43 (5): 621–35.

European Scientific Advisory Cooperative on Phytotherapy. *Monographs on the Medicinal Uses of Plant Drugs.* Exeter, UK, 1997.

Falconi, D. *Earthly Bodies and Heavenly Hair.* Woodstock, NY: Ceres Press, 1998.

Fischmann, SH et al. "Changes in sexual relationships in postpartum countries." *Journal of Obstetric and Gynecologic Neonatal Nursing.* (1986 January-February); 15 (1): 58–63.

Fleiss, P. "Herbal remedies for the breastfeeding mother." *Mothering.* 1998 Summer; 68–72.

Garvey, MJ and GD Toolefson. "Postpartum depression." *Journal of Reproductive Medicine.* (1984 February); 29 (2): 113–16.

Gladstar, R. *Herbal Healing for Women.* New York: Fireside, 1993.

Glazener, CM. "Sexual function after childbirth: women's experiences, persistent morbidity and lack of professional recognitions." *British Journal of Obstetrics and Gynecology.* (1997 March); 104 (3): 330–5.

———. "Postpartum problems." *British Journal of Hospital Medicine.* (1997 October 1–14); 58 (7); 313–16.

Gjerdingen, DK et al. "The effects of social support on women's health during pregnancy, labor and delivery, and the postpartum period." *Family Medicine.* (1991 July); 23 (5): 370–5.

———. "A causal model describing the relationship of women's postpartum health to social support, length of leave, and complications of childbirth." *Women's Health.* 1990; 16 (2): 71–87.

———. "Changes in women's physical health during the first postpartum year." *Archives of Family Medicine.* (1993 March); 2 (3): 277–83.

———. "Changes in women's mental and physical health from pregnancy through six months postpartum." *Journal of Family Practice.* 1991; 32 (2): 161–6.

Gjerdingen, DK and D Froberg. "Predictors of health in new mothers." *Social Science Medicine.* 1991; 33 (12): 1399–407.

Goldman, AS et al, "Immunologic protection of the premature infant by human milk," *Semin Perinatology,* (1994 December); 18 (6): 495–501.

Goldsmith, J. *Childbirth Wisdom.* New York: Congdon and Weed, 1984.

Gordon, AE et al. "The protective effect of breastfeeding in relation to sudden infant death syndrome (SIDS): The effect of human milk and infant formula preparations on binding of *Clostridium perfringens* to epithelial cells." *FEMS Immunol Med Microbiol,* (1999 August); 25 (1-2): 167–73.

Hanson, LA. "Breastfeeding provides passive and likely long-lasting active immunity." *Ann Allergy Asthma Immunol,* (1999 May); 82 (5): 478.

———. "Human milk and host defense: immediate and long-term effects." *Acta Pediatrica Suppl,* (1999 August); 88 (430): 42–6.

———. "The mother-offspring dyad and the immune system." *Acta Pediatrica,* (2000 March); 89 (3): 252–58.

Hanson, LA et al. "Breastfeeding: overview and breast milk immunology." *Acta Pediatrica,* (1994 October); 36 (5): 557–61

Harper, B. *Gentle Birth Choices.* Rochester, VT: Healing Arts Press, 1994.

Hasselbalch, H. "Breast-feeding influences thymic size in late infancy," *European Journal of Pediatrics,* (1999 December); 158 (12): 964–67.

Hobbs, V. *Mother Roasting: Essential Postpartum Care.* Moonflower Birthing Supply.

Huggins, K. *The Nursing Mother's Companion.* Boston: Harvard Common Press, 1999.

Keville, K and M Green. *Aromatherapy: A Complete Guide to the Healing Art.* Freedom, CA: The Crossing Press, 1995.

Kitzinger, S. *The Year After Childbirth.* New York: Charles Scribner, 1994.

Kline, CR et al. "Health consequences of pregnancy and childbirth as perceived by women and clinicians. *Obstetrics and Gynecology.* (1998 November); 92 (5): 842–8.

Johanson, R et al. "Health after childbirth: a comparison of normal and assisted vaginal delivery." *Midwifery.* (1993 September); 9 (3): 161–8.

Lang, R. "Mother roasting." *Mothering.* (1987 Spring); 55–62.

Lawrence, PB. "Breast milk: best source of nutrition for term and preterm infants." *Pediatric Clinics of North America,* (1994 October); 41 (5): 925–41.

Leary, W. "2 healthful bacteria found to ward off diarrhea in infants." *The New York Times.* October 14, 1994.

Liedloff, J. *The Continuum Concept.* Reading, MA: Addison Wesley, 1985.

Lim, R. *After the Baby's Birth: A Woman's Way to Wellness.* Berkeley: Celestial Arts, 1991.

Loras-Duclaux, I. "Practical advice for women who want to breastfeed." *Archives of Pediatrics.* (2000 May); 7 (5): 541–48.

Louden, J. *The Woman's Comfort Book.* San Francisco: Harper, 1992.

LowDog, T. *Women's Health.* Corrales, NM: Integrative Medical Associates, 2001.

Lowinsky, Naomi. *The Motherline.* New York: Jeremy Tarcher, 1992.

Luke, B. *Maternal Nutrition.* Boston: Little, Brown, 1979.

McClure, V. *Infant Massage: A Handbook for Loving Parents.* New York: Bantam, 1989.

McGuffin, M et al. *Botanical Safety Handbook.* New York: CRC Press, 1997.

McIntyre, A. *The Complete Woman's Herbal.* New York: Henry Holt, 1994.

———. *The Herbal for Mother and Child.* Dorset, Great Britain: Elements, 1992.

Mills, S and K Bone. *Principles and Practice of Phytotherapy.* London: Churchill Livingstone, 2000.

Misri, S et al. "The impact of partner support in the treatment of postpartum depression." *Canadian Journal of Psychiatry.* (2000 August); 45 (6): 554–58.

Montague, A. *Growing Young.* New York: McGraw Hill, 1983.

Nielsen, Forman D, et al. "Postpartum depression: identification of women at risk." *British Journal of Obstetrics and Gynecology.* (2000 October); 107 (10): 1210–17.

Noble, E. *Essential Exercises for the Childbearing Year.* Boston: Houghton Mifflin, 1982.

Noble, V. *Shakti Woman.* San Francisco: Harper San Francisco, 1991.

Nofziger, M. *A Cooperative Method of Natural Birth Control.* Summertown, TN: The Farm, 1979.

O'Connor, DL et al. "Maternal folate status and lactation." *Journal of Mammary Gland Biological Neoplasia.* (1997 July); 2 (3): 279–89.

O'Hara, MW et al. "Effect of interpersonal psychotherapy for postpartum depression." *Arch Gen Psychiatry.* (2000 November); 57 (11): 1039–45.

Orlando, S. "The immunologic significance of breast milk. *"Journal of Obstetric and Gynecologic Neonatal Nursing,* (1995 September); 24 (7): 678–83.

Placksin, S. *Mothering the New Mother.* New York: New Market Press, 2000.

Prentice, A. "Calcium in pregnancy and lactation." *Annual Review of Nutrition.* 2000; 20: 249–72.

Pryor, G. *Nursing Mother, Working Mother.* Boston: Harvard Common Press, 1997.

Raphael, Dana. *The Tender Gift: Breastfeeding.* New York: Schocken Books, 1976.

Rautava, P et al. "Psychosocial factors for infantile colic." *British Medical Journal.* (1993 September 4); 307 (6904): 600–04.

Reichman, S. "Asking for help and getting it." *Mothering,* fall 1982, 97–98.

Rich, A. *Of Woman Born: Motherhood as Experience and Institution.* New York: W.W. Norton, 1986.

Righetti-Veltema, M et al. "Risk factors and predictive signs of postpartum depression." *Journal of Affective Disorders.* (1998 June); 49 (3): 167–80.

Robson, KM et al. "Maternal sexuality during first pregnancy and after childbirth." *British Journal of Obsterics and Gynecology.* (1981 September); 88 (9): 882–89.

Romm, A. *Naturally Healthy Babies and Children.* Pownal, VT: Storey Books, 2000.

_____. *The Natural Pregnancy Book.* Freedom, CA: The Crossing Press, 1997.

_____. *Vaccinations: A Thoughtful Parents Guide.* Rochester, VT: Inner Traditions, 2001.

Rowe, L et al. "Mother's emotional needs and difficulties after childbirth." *Australian Family Physician.* (1996 September); 25 (9 Supplement 2): S53–58.

Russell, R et al. "Assessing long-term backache after childbirth." *British Medical Journal.* (1993 May 15); 306 (6888): 1299–303.

Ryding, EL. "Sexuality during and after pregnancy." *Acta Obstetrics and Gynecology Scandinavia.* 1984; 63 (8): 679–82.

Saurel-Cubizolles, MJ et al. "Women's health after childbirth: a longitudinal study in France and Italy." *British Journal of Obstetrics and Gynecology.* (2000 October); 107 (10): 1202–09.

Sears, M and W Sears. *The Breastfeeding Book.* Boston: Little, Brown, 2000.

Shields, N et al. "Impact of midwife-managed care in the postnatal period: an exploration of psychosocial outcomes." *Journal of Reproductive and Infant Psychology.* 15: 91–108.

Small, R et al. "Depression after childbirth: the views of medical students and women compared." *Birth.* 1997 June; 24 (2): 109–15.

Small, R et al. "Depression after childbirth. Does social context matter?" *Medical Journal of Australia.* (1994 October 17); 161 (8): 473–77.

Smolin, L and M Grosvenor. *Nutrition Science and Applications.* New York: Harcourt Brace, 1997.

Spain, V. "Home alone with the new baby." *Mothering.* Fall, 1984: 58–59.

Speer, CP and H Hein-Kreikenbaum. "Immunologic importance of breastmilk." *Monatasschr Kinderheilkd,* (1993 January); 141 (1): 10–20.

Trickey, R. "The herbal treatment of hormonally induced mood changes." *Journal of the American Herbalists Guild.* 2001, vol. 1, no, 1; 30–40.

_____. "The herbal treatment of hormonally induced mood changes." *Journal of the American Herbalists Guild.* 2001, vol. 2 no. 1; 19–28.

Tulman, L and J Fawcett. "Recovery from childbirth: looking back 6 months after delivery." *Health Care Women International.* (1991 July–September); 12 (3): 341–50.

Villalpando, S and M Hamosh. "Early and late effects of breast-feeding; does breast-feeding really matter?" *Biol Neonate.* 1998; 74 (2): 177–91.

Vissel, J and B Vissell. *Models of Love.* Aptos, CA: Ramira Publishing, 1986.

Walker, LO. "Weight and weight-related distress after childbirth: relationships to stress, social support, and depressive symptoms." *Journal of Holsitic Nursing.* (1997 December); 15 (4): 389–405.

Weed, S. *Wise Woman Herbal for the Childbearing Year.* Woodstock, NY: Ashtree Publishing, 1986.

Wertz, R and D Wertz. *Lying In: A History of Childbirth in America.* New York: The Free Press, 1977.

Whitaker, N. "Premenstrual syndrome and postpartum depression: what they are, what they do, and what you can do about them." *Mothering.* Summer 1983; 27–34.

World Health Organization. *Protecting, Promoting, and Supporting Breast-feeding: The Special Role of Maternity Services.* A joint WHO/UNICEF Statement, 1989.

Xanthou, M et al. "Human milk and intestinal host defense in newborns: an update." *Advanced Pediatrics,* 1995; 42: 171–208.

Yellis, MB. "Human breast milk and facilitation of gastrointestinal development and maturation." *Gastroenterologic Nursing,* (1995 January–February); 18 (1): 11–15.

Zinn, B. "Supporting the employed breastfeeding mother." *Journal of Midwifery and Women's Health.* (2000 May–June); 45 (3): 216–26.

Index